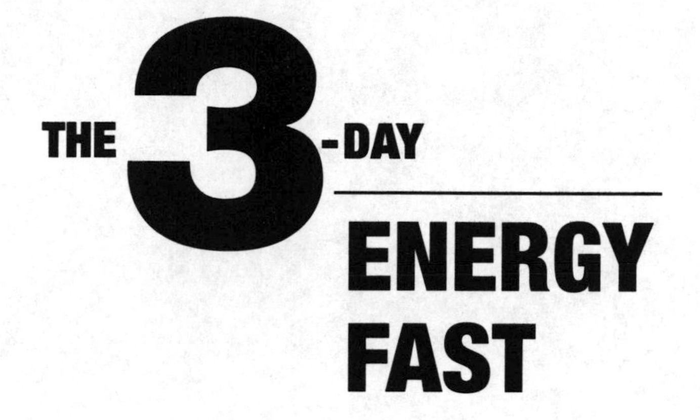
THE 3-DAY
ENERGY
FAST

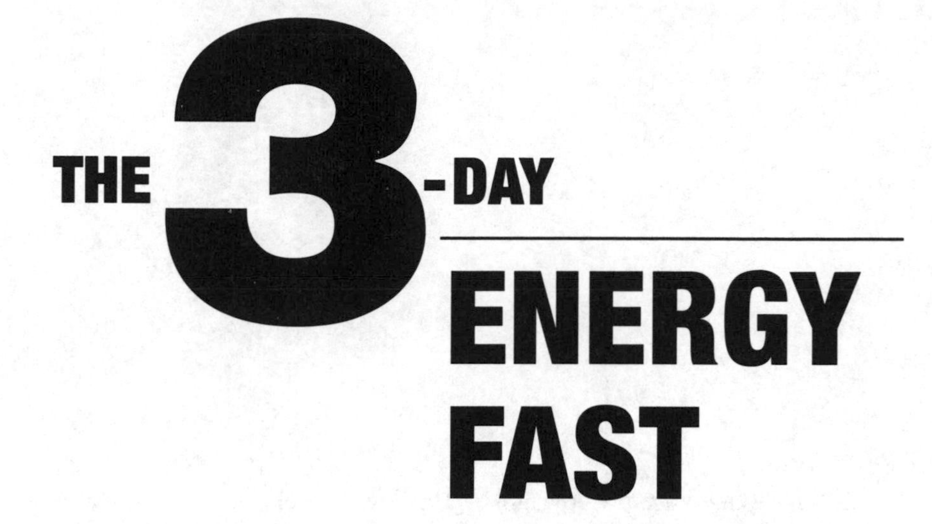

CLEANSE YOUR BODY,
CLEAR YOUR MIND,
AND CLAIM YOUR SPIRIT

Pamela Serure

HarperCollins*Publishers*

HarperCollins books may be purchased for educational, business, or sales promotional use. For information please write: Special Markets Department, HarperCollins Publishers, Inc., 10 East 53rd Street, New York, NY 10022.

FIRST EDITION

Designed by Nancy Singer

Serure, Pamela.

The 3-day energy fast : cleanse your body, clear your mind, and claim your spirit / Pamela Serure. — 1st ed.

p. cm.

ISBN 0-06-017491-9

1. Fasting—Health aspects. I. Title

RM226.S44 1997

613—dc21 96-47957

---

97 98 99 00 01 ❖/RRD 10 9 8 7 6 5 4

For Nancy, whose patience, unyielding love, support, and spirit have helped me manifest my vision and taught me to ground it. I thank you, for without you none of this would have come to pass.

And for Sage, my beautiful dog, who constantly teaches me the true meaning of meditation and how to beach walk.

FASTING

There's hidden sweetness in the stomach's emptiness.
We are lutes, no more, no less. If the soundbox
is stuffed full of anything, no music.
If the brain and the belly are burning clean
with fasting, every moment a new song comes out of the fire.
The fog clears, and new energy makes you
run up the steps in front of you.
Be emptier and cry like reed instruments cry.
Emptier, write secrets with the reed pen.
When you're full of food and drink, an ugly metal
statue sits where your spirit should. When you fast,
good habits gather like friends who want to help.
Fasting is Solomon's ring. Don't give it
to some illusion and lose your power,
but even if you have, if you've lost all will and control,
they come back when you fast, like soldiers appearing
out of the ground, pennants flying above them.
A table descends to your tents,
Jesus' table.
Expect to see it, when you fast, this table
spread with other food, better than the broth of cabbages.

—Rumi, enlightened Sufi scholar and teacher
1207–1273

Contents

Acknowledgments

I have been enriched, encouraged, and enlightened by the following people in my life. My heart belongs, in part, to each of them.

My mother and father, who always told me I could do anything in life, and now that I've almost done everything, for letting me know I would never fail, with special love and thanks for your constant love and belief.

Jeff and Toni, who believed and invested in the idea to help bring it to a reality.

Lizz, for juicing, and juicing, and juicing over and over again.

Donna K.—my beach rock buddy—for inspiring me, for arriving like an angel at the right time with the right questions, for a cashmere cushion out in the world, and for your constant support.

Barbara Lowenstein, Eileen Cope, and Madeline Morel, for being the goddesses of the publishing world.

Diane Reverand, for beaming in the vision.

Steven Carter, who shared my soul with me on the path in coming to tell this story; and Julia Coopersmith, who sharpens it, tweaks it, and sculpts it into final art.

Carolyn Conger, for the ultimate rebirth and drumming for my new spirit.

Brugh Joy, for inducting me into the true meaning of my life.

Kamala Hope Campbell, for helping me remember the path I was on.

Melinda Blau, for guiding me, chiding me, and most of all for being family.

Barbara Biziou, my cactus buddy, for making our friendship a true ritual and being there for all the changes.

Jennifer O'Day, for giving poetry and song to my new life.

Linda Horn, for sharing your genius and strength.

Lynn Kohlman, for transforming the spiritual into the visual.

Oz, who always kept my motor running and my juices flowing.

Tesh, for helping me transform my body and giving me the strength I needed.

Faith Popcorn, for seeing me in the future.

Steven Weiss, for sharing the art of business.

Stefanie Sacks, for making sense.

Robin Bonder and Meredith Israel, for taking all the calls, finding it when it couldn't be found, and for helping me look good at a moment's notice.

Beth M., Vibeke, Karin, Marybeth, Nancy, Judy, Holly, Debby, Melanie, Philip, Kavi, Sean, Camille, Rick, and all those East Healers who have worked their energy on me, supplemented me, elevated me, beautified me, massaged and manicured me, and most of all kept encouraging me to keep going.

The D.K. Beauty Group for providing me with their creative laboratories and creating a beautiful road show.

The HarperCollins team—Meaghan, David, Pam, and Steven—for their enthusiasm and commitment to me and the project.

And special Oms to:

Teddy, Beth, Hymie, Gloria, Patti, Gaby, Susie, Julie, Emily, Marnie, Reggie, Carla, Deborah, Jackie, Millie and Harry, Dr. Ash, Robin, Valerie, Niro, Eugenia, Doru, Kathy, the Banana girls, Carol, Tanya, Nicki, Eugene, Arcona, Ruth Ann, Patty C., Kevin, Michael, Judi, Valda, Paula, Patrice, Janet, Elizabeth, William, and the so many others in my life who have brought me up to this point. You are here always in my words, in the action I will take, and the service yet to be performed.

To everybody who worked with me at Get Juiced: Guy from Peter's Fruit, Wayne for balancing the chaos, Maria, my cooking soul mate, and everyone from the beginning whether it was a day, month, or season: Thank you for passing the bucket, pouring the juice, squeezing the fruit, prepping, delivering, cutting, serving, and most of all cheerleading me on. To all the Customers and Fasters of Get Juiced for really telling me what they wanted and how they felt, and for making the call very clear.

To Spirit, who every day creates the energy and faith within me and all the grace that surrounds me. I am deeply grateful.

Foreword

by Donna Karan

I hadn't been feeling great for a while and, after talking to a fellow passenger on the seaplane one day, decided to follow up on his advice about this wonderful new juice fast. I picked up the phone, called Pam and said, "I'm Donna Karan—I've got a week, what can we do?" Pamela told me to unplug my phone, my fax, and my family—and the work began.

Believe it or not, a glass of juice changed my life. The following week entailed fasting, meditation, breathing, yoga, and using my journal as a method to continue the dialogue of my journey and maintain the cleansing. I was cleaned out, calmed down, and cleared up, and prepared to continue the process as a way of life.

Meeting Pamela was stepping into a new and different phase. At the same time, it meant my entering a period of reflection on many aspects of my life. Pam helps promote the creation of a lifelong journey of nurturing the mind, body, and spirit and provides the understanding of what this all takes—*she has been there,* like each of us, experiencing the daily pains we go through or put ourselves through. Coming from the chaos of the city, she did not lose her creativity along the way; instead, she put it in a place where she discovered her own peace.

I know what she has done for me and I can only imagine what the book will do for everyone else. To my friend Pamela, someone who has helped to guide me on the path and continually supports me on my journey. I thank you.

Foreword

by Richard N. Ash, M.D., Medical Director, The Ash Center for Comprehensive Medicine

I began my medical career as a conventional physician specializing in internal medicine. I never realized the true value of "alternative" medical treatment until I became toxic to foods and chemicals that were causing severe arthritic pain resistant to standard medical therapy. I soon discovered that natural remedies, including various vitamin, mineral, and nutrient replacements combined with less processed, more alkaline foods, were more effective than drugs and didn't have side effects. As a result, I have changed my practice completely by using alternative therapies that get at the cause of the problem, rather than merely suppressing symptoms with drugs. Our consumption of refined sugar, and processed foods with a host of additives to enhance shelf life and appearance, and foods contaminated by pesticides, is, in large measure, responsible for many diseases including cancer, heart disease, allergy, and arthritis.

Throughout my research for the most effective cutting edge therapies today, I have found that to remain healthy in this toxic world, one must be actively involved in and knowledgeable about a variety of methods that lower the body's toxic burden, and give it the basic building blocks and necessary internal and external environments to heal itself.

In this book, Pamela shows you that the way we move, the kind of exercise we get, the way we breathe and think, and the way we adapt to stress in our lives play significant roles. These are the particular aspects of our lives which we can influence by our actions and attitudes.

Pam does a beautiful job of walking you through her three-day detox-cleanse step by step, with juicing, guided meditation, yoga, and deep breathing, all of which are invaluable to enhancing one's journey to optimal health.

Congratulations to Pamela and her publisher for having the foresight to produce this much-needed book.

Your health is your most important asset, and the fast, dietary guidelines, ideas, exercises, and suggestions presented in this book are not intended to replace the services of a trained health professional. If you have, or suspect, any health problems (e.g., diabetes) or any other medical condition, please consult with your medical doctor before trying the suggestions, diet, procedures, and exercises in this book. If you experience any unusual symptoms while on the fast described, please consult your medical doctor. Any applications of the fast, exercises, suggestions, or procedures set forth in this book are at the reader's discretion. If you are taking any medication, please confer with your medical doctor before attempting this fast.

Introduction

Real healing is a powerful experience. Healing is an act of kindness. Healing is an act of caring. Healing is an act of love and healing is a spiritual experience. When we heal the body, we are healing the psyche, and we are healing the spirit. The three are inseparable.

Every single one of us is holding on to some kind of emotional, physical, or spiritual pain. That's why we all need healing. Many of you reading this book may feel that you are holding on to so much pain that you no longer feel connected to anything—not even the person you are, or the person you could be. I certainly understand this feeling. For many of us, our pain is an all too real manifestation of the toxic mesh that separates us from the center of our being and the source of our energy and strength. That's why we feel as though we have no fuel or juice left for life. We are depleted, worn out, edgy, angry, and sad. This is what it feels like to be toxic.

- When you feel empty, it's tempting to try to console yourself with the wrong kind of food. We eat fatty food, sugary food, as well as food that's been processed, chemically preserved, and treated with pesticides and fungicides.
- We are emotionally toxic—filled with depression, anxiety, and a sense of being out of control. Stressful jobs, high-pressure lifestyles, difficult families, and disappointing personal relationships have pushed all of our buttons. Often we've led lives with such dramatic highs and lows that we can no longer "metabolize" or deal with our emotions.
- We are environmentally toxic because the air and the water in the places we work, live, and breathe is filled with chemicals and gases that range from unpleasant to poisonous.
- We are spiritually toxic because we've stopped connecting to a higher power. Our spirits have been exposed to so much negativity from the outside world that we feel as though we can no longer have faith in anything or anybody, least of all ourselves.

Whether it's something you ate, something you felt, something you believed, or something you breathed, chances are you have "ingested" way too much harmful stuff. What goes in is supposed to come out, but it's not always that simple. Many toxins that enter the body, the spirit, or the mind don't leave that quickly.

Maybe you can't see them, but that doesn't mean they aren't there. Even if you can't see them, you still feel them every day. You feel them as moods of fatigue, anxiety, illness, anger, and depression. You feel them as headaches, backaches, rashes, and raw nerves. They deprive you of your sleep, or they make you sleep too much. They deprive you of your strength, your stamina, and your passion for living.

It's time to do something back. It's time to take back your energy, reclaim your body, heal your psyche, and rekindle your spirits. I don't want to say that any one thing will save your life, because I don't think that is possible unless you're drowning, and somebody runs into the water with a life preserver. But I do believe there are many things that can assist in changing and transforming our lives so that when we look back, we know when we have experienced a pivotal point. For me, "getting juiced" was one of those magical transformers. I think the program I have developed can do the same for you.

For me, life detox means being able to find balance, enter back into your own spirit, and find a sense of "newness." Often, I will join new clients on the three-day program. Each time I feel as though I also have three special days to reinvent myself and become new. Everybody likes those makeovers where you go and do your hair, lose a little weight, and buy some new clothes. The problem with these makeovers is that they address only what's happening on the outside. Inside, the cells are doing the same old thing.

The whole key to personal transformation starts on a cellular level. It's about the rejuvenation of your cells. When we clean out and rebuild our cells they give us new messages. New cells have new meanings. New cells have new stories to tell. New cells don't follow the same old programming. So to transform and become new is to discover an inside banner that unfolds and says, "This is who I am." This is real healing. If you are ready to exchange your old tired cells and find new physical, psychic, and spiritual energy, then you are ready for the 3-Day Energy Fast.

Cleanse Your Body, Calm Your Mind, and Claim Your Spirit!

PART ONE

A PHYSICAL CLEANSING, A SPIRITUAL AWAKENING

1

"Please Change My Life"

"Something's going on with me, and I need help, can you help me?"

It was 9 A.M. on a Sunday, and the voice on the other end of the phone was Stephanie, a high-profile woman executive I hardly knew, and certainly didn't expect to hear from.

"What," I asked, "do you think is going on?"

"I don't know," she answered. "I don't know what's going on. I just know that something's going on with me and I need help. Please come over and help me change my life."

I get calls like this all the time; I even have a list of prepared questions I usually ask: What's not working in your life? Are you in the middle of a relationship crisis or breakup? Is your work giving you stress? But my callers often don't have any specific answers. Stephanie, for example, felt that she was on the wrong path in both her work and her personal life, but she didn't know why. As she was trying to describe her feelings, Stephanie told me that when she thought about her future, she felt scared, and her primary mood was one of uncertainty.

When I get phone calls like this, I refer to them as "angel calls." Whatever the initial motivation for the call, inevitably the person on the other end of the line believes that only a miracle could bring about the kind of healing transformation that he or she needs. These callers are reaching out for angels.

Now, I want you to know that I don't think of myself as an angel. Nor do I think of myself as a sage or guru. I think of myself as a woman who understands all too well the motivation behind these calls for help because I have been there. What I do now is work with people by showing them how to cross the bridges that are separating them from their lives. The techniques I use are both simple and profound: juice-fasting, meditation, and ritual. I love doing this because I know that this threefold spiritual process has the power to transform your spirit and help heal your body.

I have a passion for healing because for more years than I care to remember I was the one who was searching for angels; I was the one who wanted miracles and transformation. This spiritual process saved me and helped me cross the bridge in my own life.

WELLNESS IS A SPIRITUAL ACT OF SURRENDER

People typically start out confused about exactly what the combination of juice-fasting, meditation, and ritual will do for them. The program is a spiritual jump-start into a new system and a new way of being. It's like learning a new language, which gives you a new and better way to be in touch with your own life.

Fasting is not a matter of willpower. What fasting really requires is a deepening of faith and the capacity to let go, surrender to, and trust in who you are and what you can be. What carries you through a fast is your spirit not your willpower. This process asks you to surrender and give up who you are in exchange for who you can be and what can happen. By surrendering this deeply, you begin to stretch your spiritual muscles. As sages, mystics, and saints have understood for centuries, fasting is a spiritual process on the path to growth and transformation.

LEARNING TO "LET GO" IN MY OWN LIFE

Eight years ago, I was doing product development for my own company. I was stressed out, maxed out, and my juices were tapped out. I didn't feel well, and I was taking an enormous amount of medication for headaches. And then one day—not any special day—I began feeling really strange. Not well, not sick—just strange. I couldn't leave my bed, and everything was hazy.

Later that evening the room began to illuminate. This blue-white light entered the room as a tunnel appeared before me. A dear friend of mine had died of ovarian cancer a year before; she was standing there waving to me. I was so happy to see her. I began to feel really light and euphoric, most of all not sick, but well—well as I'd never felt before. It was really peaceful as my body started to glide up toward the light. Then I saw my grandparents. We were all so happy to see one another.

For whatever those moments were, I experienced complete grace—until I looked down and saw myself on the bed. There I was, this gray, green-complexioned version of myself. Just as I began to understand that my spirit had left my body, friends came into the room. They were screaming, crying, and administering CPR. I knew at that moment that leaving then wouldn't give my life the integrity I had wanted for it. It just didn't feel as though I had done what I was supposed to do. Once I had that thought, I was back in my body. And everybody around me jumped.

After that, I spent weeks in the hospital trying to get off the medications. It was a very painful experience because the process was causing seizures. No one thought I would ever be able to get off medication; if I survived, they were certain I would be on medication for the rest of my life. I was determined that the seizures would end; that this wasn't going to happen to me. And I said no, I'm not taking anything.

Through this whole period I felt as though I was getting messages. I had dreams, thoughts, and feelings that started to become imbued in my being. This truly was my spiritual awakening. When I finally got to go home from the hospital, I was so totally atrophied, I could barely walk down the block. I would put an inspirational tape into my Walkman—Bernie Siegel, Louise Hay, Marianne Williamson—and I would start trying to walk. One day I could walk only a block. Then two. I lived near the pier in New York, and I remember one spring day I was finally able to walk to the pier. But I didn't know how I was going to walk back.

For a long time my physical, my emotional, and my psychic well-being were compromised. I began to learn to scrutinize everything that went into my body. I had to examine what I was eating. I had to examine what I was drinking. I had to examine my relationships, and I had to examine what I was feeling about the people in my life. I had to examine my work and what I had been doing to make a living, and I had to examine what I was thinking. Suddenly, I could take nothing for granted. Try to imagine what it would be like to put your entire life under a microscope and come face to face with every single decision you make every moment of every day. You look at each piece of food, and wonder "Is this killing me?" You look at every piece of fabric in your home and on your body and you wonder "Is this killing me?" You look at every interaction you have at work, every interaction you have with your family, and every interaction you have with your friends, and you wonder "Is this killing me?"

It was at this point in my life that I began to understand what it meant to be toxic. It was terrifying. I realized that if I was going to heal, it wasn't going to be because of my willpower, or my ability to give up meat or caffeine. I needed to surrender.

WHAT ABOUT YOU?

Fasting, meditation, and ritual aren't just about physical health. You don't have to be flat on your back to want to remove the toxic elements in your life and feel renewed. Maybe you want to break up a relationship or leave your job. Maybe you want to start a diet or even a new business. Maybe there are important decisions you need to be making at this time in your life, or maybe you feel that you are finally ready to change your life. The 3-Day Energy Fast can help you reach your goals.

If you wake up in the morning with a hangover, it's easy to figure out that this is not the day to make essential decisions in your life. The truth is that this is exactly what most of us try to do every day—we try to make important decisions, and we try to live full lives, but we are always battling toxic hangovers. We rarely have the good energy we want and need.

Can you relate to any of these people?

- Ian, who has a very stressful job, has eating habits that are just plain bad. Since he goes to a gym regularly, and has even starting taking Tai Chi, Ian thinks of himself as someone who tries to take care of himself. Nonetheless, there are too few fruits and vegetables in Ian's diet. He consumes way too much meat and dairy products; and he loves all sweets—cookies, candy, and cherry danish, just to name a few. Whenever Ian is really upset at work, he grabs a handful of M&M's and starts chewing. This makes him feel better—temporarily. Ian doesn't know it, but his eating habits—combined with the stress in his life—are turning his system acidic. All of this makes it almost impossible for him to see his life with any clarity. There are many toxic components in Ian's life, but he thinks he's just tired and stressed. How about you? Do you have unhealthy food relationships that are combining with stress to wear you down?
- Karen is in terrible conflict over her relationship. Should she leave her partner? Should she see a couples counselor? Should she wait and hope that something will change? The conflict in her life is consuming too much energy and leaving her exhausted. In the meantime, her friend Gary is in serious conflict over his career. Should he try to change his field? Does he dare ask for a promotion at his current job? Should he go back to school? Did his parents' wishes dictate and carve out his career. Whose life is he leading anyway? His problems and the possible solutions keep bouncing around in his brain. Karen and Gary are both emotionally toxic with indecision. Do you sometimes feel conflicted, torn in two

directions, and stuck in toxic patterns like Karen and Gary?

- Mara can't open the window in her office and it makes her crazy. It is also giving her headaches and a chronic sinus infection. Some of her coworkers laugh at her, but she is not the only one in her building getting headaches, and she is not the only one complaining about the air-conditioning and the heating system. Some of her friends at work are getting rashes they can't explain. Mara and her coworkers are environmentally toxic. Are there things in your home or work environment that are making you sick—the air, the rugs, the drapes, cleaning chemicals? What about your clothes, or the lotions, potions, and medicines you put on your body?
- Alex tells his friends that he is spiritually bankrupt. He says it to make them laugh, but deep inside he knows it isn't a joke. It scares him. Alex seems to have so much going for him—he is good-looking, smart, successful—but he struggles to make meaningful and lasting connections with people, with work, and with the world. Alex is spiritually toxic. Does your life feel "flat"? Do you struggle to find things that make you feel truly happy and your life feel meaningful? Have the toxins in your life overwhelmed your faith?
- Sarah loves comfort food like ice cream, melted cheese, rice pudding, and buttered toast. She loves the way these things satisfy her as midnight snacks and she loves the way they soothe her every time she gets off the phone with her overly critical mother or has a disagreement with her overly dependent significant other. What Sarah doesn't know is that she has food allergies—she just thinks she suffers from constipation and raw nerves. Sarah is caught in a vicious cycle, trying to soothe toxic emotions with toxic remedies. Do you feel caught in your own toxic loop?

Ian, Karen, Gary, Mara, Alex, and Sarah have a lot in common. They all want a fresh start. They want to feel more alive, more spiritual, more complete, more content, and more in control of their lives. All of them want to feel renewed and replenished; all of them *want* to do good things for themselves, yet they are all filling up on some very toxic stuff.

WHAT'S YOUR STORY?

Do you roll out of bed every day, roll into work, and roll into your food? Do you have the same old fights with your partner and the same old ups and downs with your career? Do you go to sleep most nights asking yourself, what is going on? Are you so weary that life no longer feels like a surprise, full of excitement? What is it that you want in your life right now? What do you need that you aren't getting? What feels unhealthy? What feels incomplete? What feels missing? What feels in need of change? And why do you think that the 3-Day Energy Fast might be your answer?

People make the decision to go on a meditational juice fast for all kinds of reasons, and no one reason is any better or worse than the others. Before you make your decision, I think it's really important to know *your* reasons. When we approach things with a sense of clarity and intentionality, we bring a lot more power with us. And that brings results. No matter what your reasons are, the decision to fast and detox is an act of courage. The rewards are extraordinary, but the challenges are there too. Understanding your motivation from the very beginning will keep you focused, and being focused will keep you strong.

Does any of this sound like you?

"I need more energy. I'm tired of being tired all the time."

"I want to feel empowered by my life, not wiped out by it."

"I want to kick-start a diet, and I want to change the way I eat. I want to be kinder to my body, but I'm afraid I don't have the discipline."

"I want to feel more in control, and I want to make decisions I feel good about."

"I'm scared to let go of things, even when I know they're not good for me."

"I want to simplify and purify my life. I've filled my life with stuff that doesn't make me *feel* full."

"I want to find a more spiritual path."

"I want to be able to give to myself and others."

I WANT TO BE THE PERSON I'VE ALWAYS KNOWN I COULD BE

If you are like most of the people I know and work with, this is probably your deepest wish. You may have already tried lots of different ways to connect to your core and find energy, aliveness, and peace of mind. You may have done the gym thing, the diet thing, and the shopping thing. You've probably read a lot of books and talked to a lot of people. You may have attended a whole bunch of seminars, and even consulted the stars for guidance. I've done it all too . . . and then some. Healing has been my passion for a very long time; the truth is, I can't think of a single stone I have left unturned in my quest for health and wholeness. After so many left turns, right turns, wrong turns, and U-turns, it was fasting and detox that gave me the kick-start into new life that I so desperately needed.

Although deep down, every single one of us wants to feel renewed and whole, more often than not wellness and well-being elude us. Maybe right now you can't change your past, no matter how much you regret some of the things you may have done to your body, your psyche, and your spirit, but you *can* change your present. You can do something right now that will make a major difference in your life.

Getting calm, getting clear, and getting clean. Let's talk about these goals for a minute. Everyone likes the idea of being calm. Who doesn't want to wipe away anxiety and depression? Clear also sounds good. Wouldn't it be great if you were making all your decisions from a place where you felt centered, balanced, and in control. But clean is another matter. When I talk about clean, I'm talking about an internal state of well-being with emotional, physical, and spiritual systems that work together and support each other. I'm talking about a new dimension of health and vitality that comes from working deep within your body to detoxify and purify the vital systems that keep you alive, energized, and productive.

I'm talking about cleaning the liver, kidneys, intestines, colon, and other vital organs, cleaning the bloodstream and the lymphatic system, and clearing away dead and diseased cells that have been lingering for way too long. But I'm also talking about cleaning out your emotional systems—cleaning out stress, cleaning out your conscience, erasing self-defeating old tapes, letting go of anger, and letting go of grief.

SOMETIMES YOU HAVE TO TAKE ALL THE OLD THINGS OUT TO CREATE SOMETHING NEW

"Out with the old. In with the new." That's the battle cry of detox. Detox is the ultimate spring-cleaning. Detox means getting into every single "closet" in your body, including all of your emotional closets, and every single box that is in each closet. It means pulling everything out and tossing all the stuff that isn't good for you. It means getting in, cleaning up, and clearing out your system to make room for something fresh, new, and healthy.

Most of the changes we try to make in life are changes that start from the outside, and try to work their way in. A new sweater looks pretty, and we hope it will lift our spirits. A new job pays more money, and we hope it will improve our self-esteem. A new relationship looks exciting, and we hope it will give us a fuller life. A big hamburger looks rich and juicy, and we hope it will make our life feel just as rich and juicy. Detox, on the other hand, is a very different kind of animal.

Detox works from the inside out, helping you connect to your center. And if that wasn't enough, something else amazing starts to happen when you detox on such a deep level. The more healthy and alive you feel deep inside, the more your "outsides" start to mirror those feelings. A cleansing process that started at your inner core starts to show itself on the surface too. And I'm not just talking about smoother skin and lustrous hair. All kinds of things start to change. As you clean out the body of its accumulated toxins, you also start cleaning out old habits, old patterns, old ways of thinking, old ways of relating, old choices, old pain, old anger, old fears—all the accumulated old news that's no longer fit to print. Your "inside job" has come full circle, and the process feels as though it is nothing short of extraordinary. You are purifying you. You are making a new you.

INFINITE WISDOM

Sometimes, the healthiest thing we can do is to reinvoke sacred, time-honored traditions, like tending the body to honor the soul and spirit. I believe that we are all in a powerful and very exciting new time. That's one of the reasons that the process of cleansing is so important to me. If we truly are the vehicles of our destiny, then the spirit within us must be able to speak with its own true integrity. The time has come when each of us has the opportunity to be everything we were meant to be.

Throughout the ages, ascetics and holy men and women have known that fasting is a process of purification that aligns you with your spirit. Fasting is a very spiritual process that encourages you to stop what you're doing, slow down, and bring your thoughts inside. Fasting is a powerful way to come into your true essence without any disturbance from outside energy. When you fast, your body meets you. This is a beautiful way to cleanse, purify, and align with your true self. Fasting renews the spirit as well as the body. I truly wish that we could all give up the search for quick fixes and introduce this beautiful and lasting process into our lives.

There is an art to being a calm, clear, spiritual being. Three days of juice-fasting, ritual, and meditation gives a sense of that art. It gives you the opportunity to stop and listen to what you need to hear. Emotionally, the fasting process itself quiets you down. Don't we all need that? We are so over-communicated right now—we phone, we fax, we FedEx—it's too much. We're not computers. We don't have a mechanism that can process all that we have to take in during the average day. All that movement, all that confusion, all those people. Spiritual fasting stops the noise, and enables you to be with yourself in a very different way.

I understand that when you're tired and hungry, sometimes you really think you need that piece of chocolate. Well, when you fast, you stop getting that kind of message. Fasting stops the cravings. Here's why: Inside each of us there are emotional places and spaces that feel deprived, undernourished, and needy. Fasting helps you understand what you really need to fill those empty spaces. Fasting will help you to stop wanting to fill these empty spaces with food or compulsive activities.

When we use food, or alcohol, or any substance to subdue our emotions, these emotions get stuck inside. Too often we bury these emotions with food. The fasting ritual allows you to see and deal with those emotional empty spaces. By lightening up, you can let go of emotions that are not only making you hungry, but also making you sick.

I, for example, have a tendency to want to rush around and do things. That's one of the ways I fill my empty spaces. Fasting helped me sit still. How about you? Are you content to wake up in the morning and just "be"? Or do you feel lost when you don't have anything to do?

Fasting will help you be very still and listen for the messages that tell you what you *really* should be doing with your life. When your body and spirit are in alignment, there is clarity and balance. Suddenly your choices become very clear. The future doesn't look so scary, and the past isn't full of regret.

FASTING AND DETOX: WHAT'S THE CONNECTION?

To go on a fast is to give your digestive system a vacation. Who needs vacation? You do. And here's why: In a toxic world, your digestive system is working way too hard. If you eat three meals a day, that means new arrivals are showing up in your digestive system three times a day to be processed, repackaged, and moved on. If you eat four or five times a day, or if you eat all day long, your system barely gets a break. Your liver is working overtime, your stomach is working overtime, your kidneys are working overtime, your intestines and colon are working overtime. It's exhausting.

There's a reason many big companies start young hopefuls in the mail room. The mail room is the dumping ground—a place of endless work, and almost no acknowledgment. Well, that's what your digestive system is—it's your mail room, your dumping ground. Only you're the one who is doing the dumping, and you're probably doing it at least three times a day. Sure, there's a lot of good stuff that you're bringing in, but there's also a lot of "junk mail"—bad food, and various "indigestibles" that can be totally toxic in your system. But you're the one in control here. You have the power to stop the dumping and honor your system, even if it's only for a few days, by going on a fast.

Now here's the really good news: When the dumping stops, something else starts—something truly wonderful—and it starts almost immediately. That "something" is detox. No longer burdened by an overstuffed "IN basket," your digestive system can take a rest. It isn't long before *all* of your organs get into the act and start singing the same song—your kidneys, your liver, your lungs, your colon, your skin—all focused on a common goal: *detox*.

SHEDDING THE PAST TO FREE THE FUTURE

When the body is cleansed, the psyche and the spirit are also unburdened. First, the body feels revived. Ultimately, the psyche and the spirit are awakened. To detox emotionally and spiritually means surrendering your habits, surrendering your belief systems, and surrendering your compulsions, in other words, surrendering control. What people need to realize is that our toxins are all connected in the same way that the body, mind, and spirit are connected. If, for example, you're a woman whose weakness is chocolate cake and bad relationships, there is a connection. If you're a man who can't stop working and can't stop smoking, there is a connection. When we feel empty and needy, we tend to try to fill up the spaces to compensate. We're emotionally hungry so we reach for things that feel good for a moment. Detox helps you make sense of these connections, and then break the connections for good.

A great many of the people I've worked with have tried the fast to get energy. Energy, energy, energy. Isn't that what we all need more of? So many people feel as though they are chronically fatigued. When there is integrity and an effective working system, you will be able to find the energy you need. Food for me is not what we taste and chew, it's what it does. It's what we're supplying our body. Everything we eat supplies something to the system. Is the food you eat nourishing and energizing you? Is it balanced and giving you balance?

What we do in America is put food on top of more food, on top of more food. Every breakfast you eat is sitting on top of the dinner you ate the night before. Right now, constipation is one of the biggest complaints I hear above all. It robs people of a sense of energy and well-being. How could this not happen? We miscombine foods. We eat at ten o'clock at night, fall asleep, get up, and have breakfast. When you do that, you're sitting with a little mountain of undigested food.

Many of us are always filled with emotionally charged food. We're tense at work and we gobble down something fast, or we have a fight with a lover or friend, and then we eat ice cream. When this happens, do you really think the food we eat is being digested properly?

People are finally beginning to understand all the ways that the body acts as a warehouse for the toxins we can't metabolize or easily eliminate. For some people it's bad air; for some people it's bad feelings; for some people it's acid produced by stress or anger. For most of us, it's a very complex combination of many different things.

Detox is one of our most powerful ways of fighting back. The process cleanses, rejuvenates, and restores integrity to the cells, giving the system back its strength, its vigor, and its balance. From this place of restored balance, you feel physical strength, mental acuity, and emotional health.

FASTING AND REJUVENATION

When you cleanse emotionally and spiritually, everything about you clears out and lightens up. Suddenly, you are able to stop doing things the same way you've done them in the past. You find the strength to detox from all the "shoulds" in your life; you find the strength to detox from all of the unnecessary "wants" in your life; and you find the strength to detox from all the "fear" in your life. You clear away old anger and you clear away old pain. Old wounds heal, frayed nerves heal, and a fragile psyche becomes strong.

I often meet people who seem to "have it all" and have "done it all," yet they still suffer from a confusing sense of spiritual malaise. They have the job they've always wanted, the family they've always wanted, the house and car they've always wanted, the vacations they've always wanted, yet they are still left wanting *something*, even though they have no idea what that something is. With a healthier body and a healthier psyche, you are suddenly able to connect to your inner self in a new and powerful way. By cleaning out, you have cleared a pathway *in*. The spirit is awakened and the circle of healing is complete. Life feels more meaningful. Life feels more full. And you feel more full of life. Every single day, old cells die and new cells are formed. We've always heard that all the cells in the body are replaced within seven years, but I've read that we really replace 90 percent of the cells in our bodies in less than one year: Every five hours, the lining of your stomach is replaced; every four weeks, you have brand-new skin; every six weeks you have a new liver. Your body wants to be new. Your body wants to heal.

When the body is on "automatic pilot," our new cells are mirror images of our old cells, and they face the same battles. The detox process gives the body an extraordinary opportunity to recreate itself on the most fundamental cellular level. Eliminating toxins gives the body a chance to reprogram itself. With toxic material out of the way, new cells are unburdened from the "old programs" and a new, healthier, cleaner cell structure begins to form at the deepest internal levels.

Fasting with juice gives you the opportunity to build a new, healthier body from the ground up. Instead of creating new cells that are immediately compromised by toxins, diseases, and other burdens, you are making a new cellular blueprint with healthier, heartier cells and tissues as a base to build upon.

Rejuvenation is an inside job. The whole key to feeling renewed is in our cells. When we rebuild our cells, when we clean out our cells, they will help us create new lives. New cells have new diets that they want to eat; new cells have new exercise and meditation programs they want to follow; and new cells want to create new and better patterns and ways of being.

We can each kick-start our new cellular patterns by emptying out all the old food that is stuck in our bodies, the old ideas that are stuck in our heads, and the old behavior patterns that are stuck in our psyches. The 3-Day Energy Fast is about creating new beginnings. It's about starting over without starting from scratch.

Is My Life Toxic?

As Samantha was leaving work yesterday, she realized that she was so tired she felt numb. When she got home, she switched on the television and reached for the phone to order pizza and a Coke. While waiting for the delivery fix, she nibbled on the edges and bits of things, as though she wasn't really eating. She watched fifteen minutes of a deeply distressing news broadcast, two hours of mediocre television sitcoms, talked to two friends on the phone mostly about why none of them have satisfying relationships, took two aspirins, a decongestant, and three tablespoons of rum raisin ice cream. She used a facial scrub, some eye gel, and passed out. When she woke up this morning, Samantha didn't know how she was going to make it through another day. Samantha is thirty-three years old—much too young to feel this way.

What Samantha is facing is the same kind of "stuff" that all of us face. She's not as conscientious as she should be about the food she eats. She is living on a planet that is becoming increasingly more uninhabitable; she is forced to breathe badly polluted air. Her office environment—from the air conditioning to the computer screen, from the water fountain to the Xerox machine—is giving off bacteria or rays that the human body wasn't meant to handle.

When Samantha looks around her, what she sees looks unhealthy. Her office family seems hostile and unhealthy. Her own family seems dysfunctional and unhealthy. Her friends seem neurotic, obsessive, and unhealthy. Her boss seems "over the top" and unhealthy. Sometimes even her own life seems flat and unhealthy. It's enough to make Samantha feel sick, and many days, that's exactly how Samantha does feel. Sick.

There's no nice way to tell Samantha that her life is toxic, but it's something that Samantha needs to hear, and she needs to hear it as soon as possible. Samantha needs to know that something is terribly wrong with this picture she calls her life, and that she is seriously compromising her health and future. What is it about *your* world that is toxic right now? Does it look and feel a lot like Samantha's? Is it different, but still very toxic? Toxicity has many shapes and forms, because toxins do too. Perhaps your greatest struggle is with the physical toxins in your food and your environment, or with the emotional toxins in your personal and/or professional relationships. Perhaps your struggle is predominantly a spiritual one. Most likely, it is some combination. As you are weighing the pros and cons of fasting and detox, you should take a very honest look at toxicity in all of its shapes, forms, and combinations. Samantha's story is one very powerful illustration of what it means to be toxic. I'd like to give you another powerful illustration—the story of my life.

PAMELA'S STORY

If I am going to be your guide on this journey of cleansing, you need to know more about who I am. A very tough lesson I've learned is that we all must be self-protective as well as a bit skeptical before we put our health and our hearts into the hands of anyone who says she can help. The question you need to be asking yourself right now is, "Who is Pamela Serure, and why should I trust her?" I feel that the only way I can answer that question is to tell you how I came to have trust and faith in the detox program I have developed.

In my life, there have been three fully defined and consistent themes. For many years, these three organizing themes seemed to have little to do with each other. Today, they have everything to do with each other.

The first theme revolves around my profound interest in metaphysics and spirituality. I started having psychic flashes when I was a very young girl, and I began meditating seriously when I was a teenager. As a small child, I saw an angel hovering over my bed off and on for about a year. Trust me, this was not a normal everyday occurrence for a little Jewish girl growing up in Brooklyn. I kept this experience, along with my other spiritual experiences and consuming interest in these matters, a very tightly guarded secret. For years, I was embarrassed to discuss my interest in spirituality and meditation. This interest didn't quite jibe with my outside persona or the world I lived in; I was afraid it would appear wacky or weird and complicate what was then a very ambitious career track. In other words, evangelical pursuits don't look very impressive on the résumé of a product development and marketing executive looking for work in New York City.

The second theme that dominated my life until recently was a need to achieve in the business world. Like many people in my generation, I was raised to be an achiever. As a high school senior, I was trying to decide between American University and Boston University. One night, three of my aunts came over and convinced my mother that I would quickly become a pregnant dope addict if she let me leave Brooklyn to go to college. That put an abrupt end to my dreams of leaving New York, and I ended up going to school in Manhatten.

Since I was in New York and bored with college, I became stimulated by the business world. I opened my first store in Brooklyn when I was eighteen; it was called Ruby in the Dust and sold gift items from around the world.

Although I went to college to study social work, my entrepreneurial spirit kept winning out. My first store did so well that I opened another. When I was in my early twenties I began designing jewelry; I even won a few awards. Businesswoman, with a creative bent, was my persona in the real world. For a long time, my sense of self was very wrapped up in this outside success. My background taught me that you don't walk away from success. Yet my deeper questions revolved not around money or status, but around health and happiness.

The third theme in my life reflected my recurring health problems. I was a sick kid who turned into a sick adult. I had allergies, I had bronchitis, and, by the time I was four, I had had pneumonia twice. I had asthma, I had shingles, and I was accident-prone. Everyone who knows me knows that I had a series of concussions. It was bizarre. If there was an object that could hit my head, it hit my head. People kept asking me, "What are you hitting yourself on the head about?" I would laugh; they would laugh. And I would appear to forget about it until the next time I landed in an emergency room. But in truth, I never forgot about it. I knew there had to be a reason, and I knew there was some message I wasn't "getting."

My health problems escalated to crisis proportions in the mid-eighties. Although I had already been on a conscious eating plan for some time, it seemed I was becoming even more and more sensitive to my environment. At that time I was employed in the fashion industry doing licensing for a large, thriving corporation on the cutting edge of the industry. I was about to be promoted to vice president, and I was being paid good money for traveling around the world shopping and creating product.

The job seemed tailor-made for my talents, but not for me. The only problem with it was that I was keeling over. I became short-tempered, and my long-term memory turned into short-term nothing. I had stomach cramps; I had headaches; and I started to turn a not-so-fashionable shade of yellow. I had no real appetite, but I had an inexplicable craving for this gummy spearmint candy, which I would carry with me everywhere I went. I began to hate to travel, which I used to love, because every time I got on an airplane my symptoms would become worse.

Between the stress of my job, and the stress of not feeling well, my life was in crisis. I went to a maze of doctors who couldn't diagnose the problem. There were doctors who told me I must have hepatitis, even if they couldn't find it, as well as doctors who told me that if I kept going the way I was going I was going to be very ill. As far as I was concerned, I was already very ill.

I turned to alternative health practitioners. I tried everything. I went to people who did hands-on healing, nose-through healing, and healing through the ears, as well as people who told me to wear different shades of purple and orange underwear. You name it, I did it. As an example of how desperate I was, I saw somebody who stapled magnets to my ears—a friend remarked that I was so thin that if I got too close to the refrigerator, I was going to end up hanging there permanently.

In the meantime, my office was being renovated. Every slap of a paintbrush or new piece of furniture made me sicker. The new rug finally did me in. When I said the renovation was making me sicker, the company said I was crazy. I said how can I be crazy and run a two hundred million dollar division? I asked to have the rug removed. I asked to have the furniture removed. Finally I asked to have myself removed.

You need to understand that I asked to be removed from what I thought at the time was the greatest job in the world. My sense of self was very wrapped up in this outside success. Many of my friends and family thought I was out of my mind to give up this job. Often I felt the same way. My spiritual message, however, was that this couldn't continue and that I couldn't continue. One day, I was walking down a street in the garment center, and I heard a voice say, "Pamela, this can't go on." I looked around. The only person near me was a guy selling hot dogs. Could it be that a Sabrett's hot dog vendor was my personal messenger? I laughed, but it wasn't funny.

HEALING MYSELF

Convinced that I had liver cancer, I ended up in Mount Sinai's Department of Environmental Medicine being tested for toxins. As it turned out, I was completely toxic, and my liver simply couldn't handle the onslaught. I needed to get healed.

My transformation began when I left my job and the way of life attached to it. It was the biggest act of healing I had ever done. I healed myself from not having to be successful in that way. I was going toward what I needed, even if I didn't know what the next step would be. As always, healing began with surrender.

I left the city and moved to the beach. I had always meditated, but now I got really serious and more disciplined. I walked on the beach for hours. I meditated, I did breathing exercises, I did yoga, and I practiced screaming rituals, letting my voice carry into the ocean. And I made juice—lots of juice. I didn't really know what I was going to do about my career or my future, I only knew that I needed to get juiced. And that's exactly what I did. Almost immediately, I started to recover.

As I got healthier and healthier, so did my entrepreneurial spirit. I realized that I needed to pull my interests together to create a new life for myself. I was not going back to the world that I left. What would I do? I didn't really have a master plan at the time, but the first thing I decided was that I was going to sell juice. The idea was born in my kitchen. I literally spread all the fruits and vegetables out across the kitchen counter—apples, kiwis, limes, grapes. And I would ask them, Okay who wants to go together? I was talking to fruits and vegetables. I thought I was losing it, but it really didn't matter. I had peaches and plums and strawberries. What were they going to do, call up the local newspaper? With the help of my friend Lizz, we made some wild combinations, and some perfect combinations.

Once we felt that we had a handle on the combinations that worked, our little operation moved out of the kitchen. Lizz's brother Jeff owned a restaurant in the Hamptons. He let us use the restaurant kitchen at four o'clock in the morning. We would get in there and juice up a storm. My partner, Nancy Sorkow, would process the orders, bottle all the juices, and pack them in crates. It wasn't exactly Snapple yet. I went from a city slicker to someone who kept farmer's hours. Delivering the juice in my little red two-seater, I would be finished with the day's work by 7 A.M.

Boy, even without the talking, did I learn a lot about fruits and vegetables. When you handpick the tops off 1,000 strawberries for Memorial Day weekend, you become very intimate with strawberries. And when you peel 5,000 grapes off their vines, you really get to know how grapes like to be touched.

People loved the juice, and their enthusiasm strengthened my commitment. From my own experiences, and extensive research with healers and holistic practices, I already knew quite a bit about the process of healing and natural juice-fasting. So Nancy, Jeff, and I opened a little store where we began selling juice and whole foods, and I began helping people to fast using fresh juices. Eventually I realized that people wanted more, and that I had more to give.

People began coming to me for advice. I would make them the juice for three-day fasts, and I would spend time with them, and meditate with them, and walk with them on the beach. People would come to me after a three-day fast weekend, and tell me that they felt as though they had just returned from a two-week vacation. That is when I first formalized the 3-Day Ultimate Detox program. Juice had given me back my life, and meditation, exercise, and ritual had given me a life worth living. I knew that this powerful combination could work miracles for many others.

I LEARNED ABOUT DETOX THE HARD WAY, BUT YOU DON'T HAVE TO

My story is extreme. It doesn't have to be that hard or that painful, especially if you're willing to stop right now, wherever you are in your life, and take an honest look at the "big picture," and make a commitment to self-renewal. The very fact that you are reading this book right now tells me this is what you want. That's why, before we go any further, I'd like to take a moment right here to do a brief rundown of some of the toxic material that affects you, me, and everyone else we know.

THE TOXINS YOU PUT IN YOUR BODY

The human body is a fabulous piece of machinery, but it's not supposed to be a dispose-all unit. Under the best of conditions, our bodies are being abused. Even under ideal circumstances, your body would have a difficult enough time digesting all the fat, protein, and sugar the average person eats. Much of the food we eat today isn't pure, and it's less than ideal. If you eat a spare rib at the Chinese restaurant, or a grilled chicken breast in your own kitchen, chances are that it's full of hormones and antibiotics. That's because the feed that was given to these animals contained preservatives and chemicals, which are then passed along to you. How about all the chemicals that are used to grow vegetables and fruit, not to mention the chemicals that are used to preserve produce and give it a longer life.

This is before you start loading up with your own favorite chosen toxins. Few of us have been so pure that we have never ingested or inhaled large amounts of caffeine, alcohol, or nicotine. Let's take me, for example. For most of my life I never thought of myself as someone who *really* did things that were bad for my body. As far as I was concerned, I was only a dabbler. A dabbler in sweets, in cigarettes, in cosmetics and perfumes. I liked to try new things. My intention was always pure in terms of what went into my body, but like many of you, I just didn't know better. My worst offense: smoking. I loved to try different kinds of cigarettes—European cigarettes, American cigarettes, mentholated cigarettes. It took an out-of-body experience for me to stop putting smoke into my body, but that's another story.

Let's look at some of the other ways we all process toxic material.

THE TOXIC EMOTIONS THAT STEAL YOUR ENERGY

My friend Sandy, for example, acknowledges that her biggest problem is that she can't stop obsessing about her problems. She can't stop thinking, thinking, thinking in circles that never lead anywhere except back to where she started. This is making her feel so tense that she can barely breathe. She's making no connection between what she's thinking and what she's feeling—which is making her act irrationally.

Sandy places a lot of the blame on her job, which is literally taking everything she's got. It's making her so angry and irritated that she feels as though she is holding her breath all day long. She takes one big gulp of air when she wakes up. She doesn't fully exhale again until she hits the pillow and clicks on the late night TV program of choice.

When the day in front of her hits her in the stomach, her

shoulders tense up, and she doesn't feel even the slightest bit of calm again for the rest of the day. She notices that her breathing is labored; she feels the tension in her muscles; she recognizes the pain in her body and her psyche. Sandy's emotional distress is making her emotionally, physically, and spiritually toxic. Her adrenals are always working overtime, and her body is always producing enormous amounts of acid. She's in the grip of her cravings for wheat and sugar. When she sees anything doughy or sweet, she feels as if it has her name written on it.

All our emotions, all our feelings, and all our thoughts affect the physical body. Every time you have an argument with a spouse, a lover, a friend, a child, or a parent, your body responds accordingly. When you are calm, you are able to maintain a proper acid/alkaline balance in the body. If you're anxious, worried, tense, or angry, your body will start turning everything into acid. Have you ever been so upset that you've suddenly felt weak in the knees? Acid flooding through your body contributes to this effect.

Anger, anxiety, and aggravation can and will make you toxic. The way you speak, the thoughts you have, the dreams you're dreaming, the choices you make—all of these will impact on, and, in turn, be impacted by the level of toxicity in your body. Most of all in these circumstances, like will seek like, and imbalance will prevail.

THE TOXINS THAT FLATTEN YOUR SPIRIT AND STEAL YOUR FAITH

Are any of the elements of your life stealing your spirit?

Are you living in the past? Are you living in the future? Are you living in fantasy? Or are you living in fear? Are you living for today? Are you living in a soap opera? Do you accept your life today as it is, or are you always asking what's missing? Do you know what it takes to create balance? Do you know how to "fill up" or are you so accustomed to running on empty that you no longer know the difference? How many experiences help you stay connected to your own sacred inner space? How many experiences bring you closer to a feeling of unity with nature or anything that you consider truly divine? What is your connection to a higher source? So few of us take the time or energy to give the spirit the tending that it so deeply needs. It may even sound to you as though I am speaking a foreign language right now. If it does, you should know that this is a language you desperately need to learn.

People who are spiritually toxic tend to feel as though they are unable to live in the moment, and are always looking for others or outside events to make them feel better. There is no faith, and consequently, fantasies replace real hope.

HERE A TOXIN, THERE A TOXIN, EVERYWHERE A TOXIN

- From perfume to shaving cream, from lipstick to eye shadow, we all absorb our share of potentially toxic ingredients and allergens through our skin . . . every day.
- Whether it's prescription or over-the-counter, we all take our share of medicines to make us feel better. Antibiotic, antihistamine, anti-acid, or anti-inflammatory, your system has to find a way to get those drugs out of your body.
- When I talk about the toxic workplace, I'm not describing your neurotic employer, your driven coworkers, or your hostile assistant. Not here anyway. I'm talking about inadequate ventilation systems, manmade fibers, chemicals, fumes, varnishes, paints, and synthetic wood. Take a plane trip, and the air is so bad, it takes twenty-four hours to recover. Ride the New York subway system or in a car on a Los Angeles freeway, and you know what toxic air smells like.

TOXIC SYMPTOMS MAY COME AND GO

For most of us, toxic symptoms are a group affair. Unless you're paying close attention, it's easy to forget what symptoms arrived when or how. And you're probably *not* paying close attention, especially since part of being toxic is not having the time or mental energy to attend to what you are experiencing. As each symptom appears, you try to push it away and go on. You're tired and you're not sleeping well. You have a rash, and you don't know why. You become accustomed to frequent stomachaches. Your back hurts. You feel starved, and if you're a woman, you assume it's your hormones. You're depressed and you think it's because of a relationship, or the lack of a relationship.

Can you see how easy it is to be clueless about your own body? That's where healing comes in. Healing means being willing to put it all together; it means looking at the many puzzle pieces that you have and connecting them until they form a bigger picture. This picture is the first stop on the road to self-renewal.

WHAT ARE YOUR "HOT SPOTS"?

It's time to finish putting your picture together. And that's where it's going to help to get very specific. It's one thing to feel, or even to say "I'm toxic." It's quite another to have your own list of signs and symptoms right in front of you. So, keeping all this in mind, I'd like you to look at the following sets of questions. Take your time, giving each question some serious thought, then mark your answers in the space provided.

ARE YOU IN NEED OF A PHYSICAL CLEANSING?

1. Are you putting on weight as the years go by?

   ____

2. Are you always hungry?

   ____

3. Does your body seem to want sweets and "carbs" more than it does protein?

   ____

4. When you wake up, is there a bad or metallic taste in your mouth? Does it take a while to go away?

   ____

5. Do you get frequent headaches?

____

6. Are you often cranky and short-tempered?

____

7. Is your complexion less than bright?

____

8. Do you suffer from periodic breakouts, rashes, or skin conditions?

____

9. Is your eyesight blurred?

____

10. Are you frequently constipated?

____

11. Do you get a bloated feeling after eating that takes a while to go away?

____

12. Do you experience lots of gas, belching, or heartburn?

____

13. Does it feel as though you're always "fighting something"—a cold, a sore throat, a flu, etc.?

____

14. Do you feel really vulnerable to getting sick?

____

15. Do you often feel tired even when you've had enough sleep?

____

16. Is your energy getting harder and harder to access?

____

ARE YOU IN NEED OF AN EMOTIONAL CLEANSING?

1. Do you have cravings that are hard to control (*any* kind of cravings—food, alcohol, cigarettes, sex, shopping, etc.)?

   ____

2. Do you have a hard time crying or expressing emotions? Is it hard for you to get angry or to express that anger?

   ____

3. Is food more comforting to you than human relationships?

   ____

4. Do you prefer to be alone—all the time?

   ____

5. Do you feel sad or down much of the time?

   ____

6. Do you often feel an anxious knot in your stomach?

   ____

7. Are you easily affected by other people's moods?

   ____

8. Do you need immediate gratification of all your needs?

   ____

9. Do you tend to keep old wounds open, bear grudges, hold on to your anger, or stay immersed in self-pity?

   ____

10. Does it feel as though many of the choices you make in your personal and/or professional life have become counterproductive, if not self-destructive?

    ____

11. Have you stopped believing in your future?

____

12. Is your list of regrets growing?

____

13. Are you easily disappointed?

____

14. Does it feel as if you have no frustration tolerance?

____

15. Would you rather be right than happy?

____

16. Are you always trying to "fix" or change something about yourself?

____

17. Do you never seem to feel perfectly at ease?

____

ARE YOU IN NEED OF A SPIRITUAL CLEANSING?

1. Do you feel as if you're just "surviving" your life, and not *living* it?

____

2. Does it feel as if your life has pretty much been "written" and that there isn't much to look forward to anymore?

____

3. Do you often let someone else's energy and needs direct your life?

____

4. Have you stopped trying to create or invent newness in your life?

 ___

5. Do you feel as if there is no such thing as "your destiny"?

 ___

6. Are you less and less able to be with yourself and be still?

 ___

7. Do you fill your life with activities and noise to make yourself feel full?

 ___

8. Have you given up on finding anything out there in the universe that is "bigger" than you?

 ___

9. Do you feel disconnected from any sense of purpose or meaning?

 ___

10. Do you feel as if you're on a treadmill that isn't going anywhere, but that you can't make it stop?

 ___

11. Are you always racing through your life, and never savoring any of it?

 ___

12. Do you feel skeptical about or uncomfortable with the concept of a "higher power"?

 ___

13. Do you feel as if you're carrying the weight of the world on your shoulders?

 ___

14. Is a feeling of real joy missing from your life?

____

15. Do you feel unprotected in the world?

____

16. Does life feel like something you "tolerate," but rarely, if ever, enjoy?

____

As you probably have guessed, every "yes" answer is a sign of toxicity. How many questions did you mark with a "yes"? More than four in each category, and you've earned frequent-flier miles on the 3-Day Energy Fast. Think about how each of these toxic symptoms is affecting your life right now. Is this something you want to change? Is this something you want to change *now*?

YOUR FUTURE IS ALREADY BEING REWRITTEN

I remember how I felt the first time I learned about the signs and symptoms of toxicity. I was so relieved! So many things that were scary and confusing in my life started to make sense. The good news was that I wasn't going crazy and I wasn't dying from some mysterious illness! And I wasn't the only person on the planet who felt the way I felt. The bad news was that I wasn't healthy.

Maybe you're feeling the same kind of relief right now. Or maybe you are using these checklists as a reason to get angry with yourself or pass judgment on your past behaviors. If you are, you need to *stop right here*! These checklists aren't here to make you feel bad, they are here to help you start feeling *good*. This is a book about healing, and healing begins with forgiveness. You can't change your past; you can only accept it, try to understand it, and then create a different present. And you are already doing just that.

Even as you read these pages, your future is being rewritten. Now that's a pretty big statement, but it's true. That's the beautiful thing about finally becoming *aware* that you need a life detox.

Once the news hits the stands—once you become fully conscious of what's going on—things start to change almost immediately. That's when you start doing something to become new. Believe me when I tell you that your mind, your body, and your spirit have already "taken a meeting," as they say in Hollywood, and started to reorganize at a very deep level. You may not be conscious of it yet, but the healthiest parts of you are already preparing to take back your health and your life. It's a simple truth: The very act of opening your eyes and taking a closer look at your life has already started to change your life. So, while it may not feel as if you have "done" anything, you need to know that you have already done an *amazing* thing—you have planted the first seeds of transformation.

ARE YOU READY FOR MAGIC?

What follows next is a conscious decision to take action. Right now, you may be feeling motivated. You may be feeling absolutely inspired. Maybe you think you are ready to calm your body, clear your mind, and claim your spirit. You also probably have a lot of questions about the process of fasting and detox—important questions that need to be answered before you make a decision to do *anything*. It's my turn to answer some of your questions, and attend to what are likely to be some of your greatest concerns.

Three Days: Is That Too Much to Ask?

Detox and cell renewal are the rallying cries of the era of wellness. And for good reason. The truth is that in today's world, all of us need renewal. By making the decision for detox and self-renewal, you are really deciding to help your body do the job it has always been designed to do. Committing to a three-day fast may feel like a radical decision right now, especially if you've never done anything like this before, but there is really nothing very radical about it. You are simply taking advantage of your body's natural drive toward wellness. All you will be doing is giving the process a little assistance for a few days. And that's where fasting comes in.

WHY DO WE USE JUICE TO FAST?

There are all kinds of ways to fast. The only fast I ever recommend is a juice fast, supplemented with natural springwater and mineral broths. My juice fast is not about starvation; it's about cleaning out and replenishing. The fast is very gentle and healing. I really believe that raw juice is the nectar of life. Juice is a live food, carrying vitamins, minerals, antioxidants, and enzymes to your body quickly and efficiently. Yet as far as your digestive system is concerned, raw juice is almost an "invisible" food since it requires virtually no digestion! Nutrients are absorbed and utilized with minimal work, giving your digestive system a chance to get a solid rest without making your body suffer from any kind of deprivation. What could be more perfect.

Let's slow down for a second and take a closer look at everything that your body gets when you are giving it only juice:

- You get vitamins and minerals to keep all your vital systems healthy and highly functioning throughout the fast.
- You get enzymes for cleansing and rebuilding throughout the fast.
- You get antioxidants, the natural youth-keepers that fight the aging and dangerous free radicals.
- You get liquids, to continuously flush the system and carry away toxins during the fast.

RAW JUICE IS NATURE'S SCRUB BRUSH

There's a very good reason that rejuvenation has become such a buzzword in our culture. The concept is not just a clever marketing ploy, it is a reflection of our vital needs. We have all this dead stuff inside of us that we are holding on to. Dead cells, denatured thoughts, and dried-up emotions. The details about how skin cells regenerate has created a billion-dollar beauty business. Right now, if you walk through the skin-care section of any department store, you're going to be told to exfoliate and slough off all those dead skin cells. I think that's a great idea. But what about you, at your core? The cells inside your body are where you need to start your regeneration and rejuvenation process. Raw juice will help you do this.

The fast I'll be teaching you starts in the morning with fruit juice. Fruit juices are really effective when it comes to cleansing and scrubbing deep inside the body. Fruit juices are a beautiful, powerful wash, taking away your personal dreck. They also bring the natural sweetness of life into each morning, reminding us how beautiful it is to be on this earth.

In the afternoon of each fasting day, we'll change over to vegetable juices to help rebuild. At the deepest levels of the body you'll be creating new life by building new cells, the building blocks of human life, and your vegetable juices will be an instrumental part of that.

Both fruit and vegetable juices tend to make the body somewhat alkaline. (Many people don't realize this, but even though many fruit juices are acidic before they enter the body, they quickly turn alkaline when they reach the stomach.) An alkaline system discourages the growth of harmful bacteria, as well as many other unwelcome guests. With fewer intruders to fight, the body is free to concentrate its energies on rebuilding. It's a one-two combination that has no equal.

RAW JUICE LIFTS THE SPIRITS

Fasting with fruit and vegetable juice helps you cleanse, rebuild, and introduce balance into your life. Emotionally and spiritually, drinking fresh juice inspires a lovely feeling for the richness of life. Go to a farm stand or a farmer's market and watch people's eyes as they look at the glorious freshly picked fruit and vegetables. Farm stands and markets connect you to the vitality of fresh foods, a connection that is often dulled or lost in the typical supermarket experience. Juice-fasting has the same effect. It's like living at a fabulous fresh farm stand for three days.

I have people who come to me with "emotional hangovers." Typically they're breaking up a relationship and grieving; nothing in their life feels right, nothing tastes right, and either they don't want to eat anything, or they find themselves eating everything. Fresh juices make all the difference. Juices become the sweetness in life again for them, bringing new aliveness and new hope.

If a glass of orange juice in the morning is your typical juice experience, you're in for a big surprise. There's an amazing world of fresh juices and juice combinations out there that are absolutely stunning, occasionally startling, and almost always deeply satisfying.

I'm going to teach you all you need to know about making simple but spectacular combinations of fruit and vegetable juices, along with a satisfying vegetable mineral broth that is to be sipped in the evenings.

ADD MEDITATION, GENTLE EXERCISE, AND RITUAL, AND MAGIC HAPPENS

Although juice-fasting is the cornerstone of the Ultimate 3-Day Life Detox Program, this program is more than just a fast. It is a comprehensive program offering special meditations, gentle exercises, and comforting rituals, all of which support and magnify the process of detoxification.

The Ultimate 3-Day Life Detox is a three-day retreat—a health spa for the mind, the body, and the spirit. Three days to turn the outside world off and turn in to yourself. It is a time for deep surrender and self-acceptance. A time to be fed, be cared for, and be healed. It's a time to get healthy and to get connected. A time to grow, to get strong, and to get balanced. It's a time to get smart, to get serious, and to get going with your life—the kind of life you've always needed and wanted. It is a time for transformation—the right time—now.

People often go to spas or retreats for long weekends so that they can get motivated about dieting or decision-making. That's great, but frequently when they return from these places and enter their own worlds they lose what they've learned. I don't want that to happen to you. I want you to have everything you learn from this program to keep for the rest of your life. And your own home is the place where you want to feel better for the rest of your life. That's why I think it's better to start this journey at home.

The requirements are simple. First you need to say "yes" to yourself. Then you'll need two essential tools of the trade: a blender, which is something you probably already have, and a juicer, which you may have to buy or borrow. Last, but not least, you'll need three days.

JUST THREE DAYS

Three days of your life . . . that may sound like a lot of time right now. But, once again, think about the payoffs. Think hard.

Three days to find greater energy, wholeness, and inner clarity. Three days to look and feel like the person you always knew you could be. Three days to open the passageway to transformation. Three days to start your juices flowing. It could be the wisest investment you ever make.

If you were feeling balanced right now, I know that you would not be reading this book. If you felt your life was really "working," you would be out just living it. But something isn't working. And it isn't working for *most* of us. The fact that you have come to this book says you have the willingness to try something new, to make a fresh start, and to find real health.

Our willingness to change is very beautiful. We change things so much and so often in our lives. We change our homes, we change our jobs, we change the way we dress, and we change the way we look; we change who we are to our friends, to our mates, and to our children. The very hardest change is to give to ourselves. The hardest thing for most of us to do is to say, "I deserve this, and I am giving this change to myself. This is not for my family, or my mate, or my boss . . . this is for me."

I must applaud each and every one of you who is reading this right now and thinking maybe, just maybe, I want to try this . . . maybe I could do this. The word "maybe" is the biggest word in our body. It is the word that cracks open the door, giving us a chance for a new beginning. It brings us closer to the mystery of life, the beauty of life, and the fullness in life. It is the word from which all others unfold.

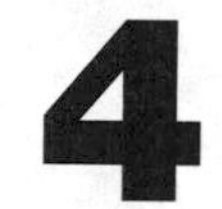

Creating a New Life Story

Barbara is deeply committed to change, and that fact alone makes her the perfect person to go on a three-day fast. Barbara has several issues that are troubling her, and fasting and meditation could help her resolve these issues. Barbara always feels that she is making the same kinds of mistakes time and time again. She would like to stop doing this, but she never has any foresight. Only hindsight.

Right now, Barbara has some major decisions she feels she should make about the direction her life should take. She realizes that when her last serious relationship ended, she never resolved her sense of disappointment and loss; in addition she is unhappy that she hasn't been able to find another meaningful relationship. Barbara's overriding complaint probably involves a sense that she has a destiny that she's not fulfilling. She feels lost; she feels as if she needs a spiritual guide, and she doesn't know where or how to look.

Isn't that how most of us feel much of the time—as if we need a spiritual guide. Don't you wish that you were doing with your life what you were meant to be doing? Don't you wish you had help making sense of your life story? And don't you believe that there really is an answer about what you should do in your life?

FINDING YOUR GUIDE

Each of us can receive the spiritual guidance we need to take the right roads and make the right decisions. All you need to do is listen to what you're being told by your higher self and let it guide you to do what it is you need to do. This may sound very complex and otherworldly right now, but it actually becomes quite simple.

Fasting and cleansing is the most direct method I know of reaching our inner being and connecting to the higher self. It's as though you are creating a temporary window to the inside. Imagine a magical message board deep inside you—a board filled with a lifetime of messages from your body, your psyche, and your spirit, just waiting to be read. This is a board with vital information about you, your life, and your destiny. For years, this board has been covered with dust and debris from the bad foods you may have eaten, the pollutants you have taken in from the air, water, and earth, and the "emotional fallout" of unfulfilling relationships, stress, and other negative life experiences. When you fast and detox, you are clearing away this dust and debris, leaving yourself more open and able to hear the messages you could be hearing. It is these messages that will become your teacher and your guide.

Some of these messages will be simple and straightforward. For example, your stomach may tell you "Carbs make me feel bloated!" Other messages may be complex and profound. For example, your psyche may tell you, "I am still furious at my father for abandoning me when I was a little girl." Some of these messages will come in loud and clear, while others may be only a mere whisper inside of you.

As you begin to listen, it may be only the loudest messages that you can hear. A typical loud message could be something like "I need more sleep every night!" If you let yourself hear these louder messages, and you follow their wisdom, you will soon invite the more gentle-voiced, spiritual messages. These are the messages that will grow stronger as you cleanse and purify, helping you find your true path, and guide you to your destiny. Over time, there is no limit to the richness of information and guidance that awaits you. The more you listen, the more you will hear. The more you believe, the more you will hear. The more you act, the more you will hear.

Messages from within, like gemstones in a deep mine, may be uncovered one at a time, or they may be found in clusters or rich veins. You never really know until you start fasting and cleansing. The one thing you can trust is that the messages are there, waiting to help you, to guide you, to care for you.

Are you ready to discover your true destiny? For some individuals, the experience can happen quickly and miraculously. Perhaps you will be one of the lucky people who has this kind of epiphany. For the majority of us, however, finding one's destiny is a process—an extraordinary, exciting process of uncovering the many messages that wait deep within, and following those messages to stay true to your path. Following your inner voice often means making changes, both big and small. For me, this incredible journey of change is what real life is all about. Everything I do in my life I do to support this journey. Nothing I have ever experienced is more inspiring, more fulfilling, and more complete. It is my hope that you too will embrace your journey and give it the status and celebration it deserves.

REDESIGNING YOUR LIFE

You won't find me listed in the Yellow Pages under "Interior Design," but when I am working with people on a one-to-one basis, I ask them to think of me as their interior decorator—the person they have hired to help them bring their beautiful house to life. The beautiful house I am referring to is the body/mind/spirit—the totality that is the individual. Together we sit down and take a close and caring look at this house. Then I help them use the information we have gathered to make important decisions about how they want to proceed.

Think about this for a moment. If you were an interior decorator hired to redecorate a beautiful house, how would *you* proceed? You wouldn't start buying furniture and rugs or choosing paint chips and tile before you knew what the rooms looked like, would you? Of course not. First, you would want to walk through that house over and over, studying it carefully and lovingly. And you would have lots of questions. What is the history of the house? What has been done to it over the years? What kind of people are living in this house? What are their tastes? What is their budget? The answers to all of these questions would give you the guidance you need to do the best job possible.

As you are about to discover, it isn't that different when you are taking on the task of cleansing and detox through fasting. From now on, I want you to think of yourself as an interior decorator, and to think of your mind/body/spirit as the beautiful house that you have decided to make your work. Before you proceed, lots of questions need to be asked and lots of information needs to be gathered. This information will be a vital source of guidance throughout your three-day fast, and hopefully, for the rest of your life. It will help you make important decisions about how you want to approach the fast, how you want to handle the three-day fast itself, and how you may want to proceed through the days, weeks, months, and years that will follow. It will also give tremendous support to those decisions. Now I know you're probably eager to get started. And sure, you could dive right in to the fast and try to "wing it" as you go. But doesn't your house deserve more love and attention than that? After all, it is the only house you'll ever have in this lifetime. I hope you will agree with me and take the time now to sit down and follow some of the simple, enjoyable exercises presented in the next few pages.

CREATING A SACRED SPACE

Writing a new life story begins by reflecting on your life in the past, and continues by opening yourself up to the future. To do this means connecting to your inner voice and allowing it to teach you about your history and guide you toward your true destiny. Making sense of your life story is a very private process and a very internal process. It isn't something you want to do while you're watching television, while you're sitting in rush hour traffic, or when you're in a room full of people. To facilitate your process, the first thing you need to do is to establish a very special and sacred place where you can dedicate your time, energy, and focus to you. This is your sacred space.

We all need a sacred space, a quiet, private place to be alone with our thoughts and our feelings; a place where we are free from disruptions, interruptions, external challenges, and internal demands. How many times have you thought "If only I could have a few minutes alone," or "If only I could hear myself think," or "If only I could take care of myself as well as I take care of so many other people in my life." Well, creating a sacred space is the first step toward making all of these wishes come true.

Your sacred space is any private little spot you can call your own. Now is the time to start thinking how you might create such a space for yourself. Is there any room in your house where you could sit and meditate and have complete privacy whenever you need it? Is there a place in your garden? Your sacred space could be a room, a portion of a room, a table, a shelf, or any space that you can claim as your own.

Your space needs to be a place where you won't be disturbed by nosy neighbors, barking dogs, or ringing telephones. If there is a phone in your space, either take it out or turn the ringer off and let your answering machine take your calls. If you live with others, maybe you can put a screen around your sacred space, or maybe you just need to make it clear that when you are in your space you shouldn't be disturbed.

For those of us who grew up in households where no space was ever our own, the idea of creating a separate, quiet space may seem very radical, if not absolutely strange. Believe me, you will get used to it very quickly; it probably won't be long before you are wondering how you have lived for so long *without* a sacred space. Are you worried about making your loved ones feel excluded? Then you need to tell yourself that no matter how much love you have for the many people in your life, there are times when you need to be able to separate from them, even if it is only for a short while. Give yourself the opportunity to make a heartfelt connection with your inner self. This connection will not diminish your capacity to give to others. On the contrary, it will strengthen it. Having a sacred space for yourself is an incredibly loving act.

SANCTIFYING YOUR SPACE

The sacred space is a place where you know you will be able to find peace of mind. If you bring all of your worries, concerns, pressures, and problems into your special space, it will not feel sacred and it will not serve you. If you bring in all of your conflicts and negativity, it will feel contaminated and it will not serve you. Once you have chosen your space, it always needs to be respected. The following exercise will help you establish and celebrate the sacredness of the special space you are going to use.

Protecting Your Space

Start by sitting cross-legged on the floor, or in a comfortable chair within your sacred space. Extend your right arm fully in front of you and point your index finger. Now, using your index finger as though it were a pencil, draw an extended imaginary circle completely around yourself. Be sure to complete the circle so it is protecting you on all sides.

Now, close your eyes and think for a moment. What have you brought into this circle today that is a source of stress, anger, frustration, worry, concern, sadness, or fear? Did you bring your monthly mortgage and credit card bills? Did you bring a memory of last night's bad date? Did you bring the list of things you need to do this week, the disagreement you just had with your sister, or the problems you're having with your child's elementary school teacher? *One by one* I want you to take each of these things in your hand, as though you could actually pick them up, and place them outside of the circle.

It is important to symbolically remove every item with a concrete physical gesture. If it is your boss, for example, imagine a tiny replica of this person right in front of you—pick him/her up and place him/her outside of the circle. Use your strength to push and keep each item outside of the circle. If they insist on hanging around the perimeter for now, that's okay, as long as they don't come inside.

Dedicating Your Space

To make your space truly sacred, it must be dedicated to you and you alone. Others may be invited to join you in spirit, but that decision is only yours to make. Right now I want you to think about all of the *positive* people in your life who, in your thoughts, you have carried with you into your sacred space. One by one, you need to imagine gently picking them up in your hands and carrying them to the outside edge of your circle. They can stay nearby, they just need to remain outside your personal boundary. In a few moments you will be inviting some of these people back in, but right now, it is important to hold on to the feeling of being absolutely alone in a space that is dedicated entirely to you. Once the only person you are thinking about within your space is YOU, and you have fully felt this separateness, you have sanctified your space.

FINDING JOY IN BEING ALONE IN YOUR SPACE

For some of us, the thought of being absolutely alone, even for just ten or fifteen minutes, is very frightening. When we don't have *any* time to ourselves, we moan and groan about it. We tell everyone it's the one thing we need . . . the one thing we crave. But when you actually get the chance to have that time, to separate from everyone in your life, even the thought of it can be overwhelming. Is it absolutely necessary to create a separate, sacred space? I think it is. Creating a place to be fully alone is one of the most powerful ways I know to invite transformation. So many of us are used to turning to the outside for comfort, for healing, and for wisdom. But it is in the process of turning *in* that the finest answers can be found.

This was a very big surprise to me at first, and may come as a surprise to you too. I love to be with people. It was sometimes hard for me to imagine that I could be my own greatest source of comfort and support. Experience has proven to me that this is true, and soon you will have that experience too.

I'm not suggesting that you are supposed to be alone all of the time, or that it's a good thing to be a loner. I'm just saying that time alone is a powerful tool for transformation. In the absence of distractions and demands, we can feel and hear more fully. In this place of aloneness we are taking the best care of ourselves. There is less fear, there is less pressure, and there is more peace.

FILLING YOUR SPACE

Now that you have created a separate and sacred space, it is time very consciously and deliberately to fill that space with things that help you feel grounded and connected. This is something that should be done slowly and thoughtfully. Try to make it into a ceremony, remembering that everything you bring into this space should have special meaning to you.

Perhaps you want to bring in photographs of people you love. A few minutes ago, you needed to usher these people out of your space, but now may be the time to lovingly welcome some of these people back. You may find that photographs of yourself, such as your favorite baby pictures, can be particularly comforting. Maybe you want some of your favorite books of poetry or art. Maybe you want lots of stuffed animals. Maybe you want toys or other playful things like art supplies. Maybe you want seashells or crystals or mementos from your childhood. I know one man who treasures an autographed baseball that his father got for him the first time he took him to a baseball game and I know a woman who has a copy of the *LIFE* magazine that was on the newsstands the day she was born. Think about what objects remind you most of the best that is in you. These are the things you want with you, to keep you company and nurture you in your space.

You want to fill your space not just with objects, but also with wonderful smells and sounds. You should be able to listen to music you love within this space (if you don't have a stereo, consider getting a small portable unit or Walkman). Scented candles, potpourri, or fresh flowers fill a space with magic. So does incense. Or perhaps you'd prefer a small set of chimes. If it soothes you, lifts your spirits, or makes you feel alive and loved, bring it into your space.

BUILDING AN ALTAR

Once you have filled your sacred space, I encourage you to create a little altar within this space. This altar is the place where you can go to have dreams and visions, and to have these dreams and visions realized. For me, an altar is a universal meeting place—a little station where you can communicate with your true essence, and with the world.

The easiest way to create an altar is to use a table (or a portion of a table), a shelf, or a corner of a floor. Since you want your altar to be special, I would begin by finding a beautiful cloth to cover the altar space. If you already have a piece of fabric that has special meaning to you, even if it's an old T-shirt or jersey, this would make an especially wonderful foundation for an altar. Your altar reflects your sense of beauty, so you want to use it to hold things that are beautiful and meaningful to you. Look at what you brought with you into your sacred space and think about which of these most reflects the best of your spiritual qualities—these would be the things you want on your altar.

Perhaps you also want to put a photograph on your altar to help anchor you—someone with whom you've studied, someone close to your heart, someone you've met in your travels, someone who opened you up to a sense of spirit, or someone who gives you a sense of safety and caring. Perhaps you have other things that anchor you, such as a special rock, crystal, amulet, or lucky charm that you carry. Place these on your altar, too. If you don't have an object like this, now would be a wonderful time to find one. Anything that connects you to your innermost self and your higher power is appropriate for your altar.

Building an altar is a meaningful way of acknowledging the existence of a higher power. Whether your higher power is God, nature, planet earth, the cosmos, or the chair you are sitting on, creating an altar is your way of saying that there is something in the universe that is bigger and more powerful than you, and that you believe that "something" is taking care of you. Building an altar is about giving up control, about surrendering. An altar involves trust and faith.

Once you have created your altar, how will you use it? Think of your altar as the place where the most important aspects of your life are brought into focus. It is the place where you will symbolically bring your most pressing issues and concerns in the hope of receiving insight, help, resolution, or healing. When you place something on an altar, you are symbolically saying that you are turning this concern over to a higher power. This is a powerful way to begin reconnecting (or connecting for the first time) to the spiritual part of your life.

You can put anything you want on your altar, and you can change it whenever you want. You can, for example, write down your fears and worries and place that paper on your altar. Or you can write down your hopes and wishes. I use my altar all the time, and I must admit that for me it has had an almost miraculous effect. When I am concerned about the well-being of friends and loved ones, I place their names or their photographs on my altar. When I wish to give thanks for something I have received, I symbolically place it on my altar. When I need to bless a new venture, I symbolically place it on my altar. Does it make a difference? Let me just say that when I was dreaming about opening a shop that would help introduce the concepts of detox and juice-fasting, all I had was the name, "Get Juiced." I wrote it down on a piece of paper and placed it on my altar. Within days, I was able to formulate a concept of what I wanted this juice business to be. My altar became like the marketing director. Every time I brought a step to the altar, it gave me the next step. Within months, "Get Juiced" had gone from a name on a piece of paper to an ongoing business.

When I was thinking of buying a house, I put the picture of the house I wanted on my altar, and then I got the house. To this day I always do it, and I tell friends and family to put their wishes on their altars. Once when I went to Florida to visit my parents, they were both in a slump. I suggested to my mother that she build an altar. "What do you mean?" she said. "We're Jewish." Nonetheless she agreed to try it. Because she was embarrassed to let anyone see it, she put her altar on a television swivel so she could turn it toward the wall so nobody else could see it. She was a closet altar person. One day she called me to say, "Pamela, I don't understand it, but everything I put on my altar happens."

If there is something you are trying to accomplish, achieve or discover, something that would really serve who you are, whether it's a new job, a new home, a new relationship, or a new life—you want to use your altar to help you and bless you. Write it out on a piece of paper in the form of a wish and place it on your altar. Ask your angels, your God, your goddesses, your animal kingdom—whatever entity or entities make sense to you—to help you achieve your wish if it is in your best interest, and for the highest good. While you are there, light some incense and a candle as a dedication. Snuff out your incense and candle, and leave the piece of paper on the altar.

LOVE LISTS

If you've never built an altar before and aren't quite sure what to place on it first, my suggestion would be to create what I call a "love list." A love list is a list of ten things that you love. Here's *my* list:

1. I love to meditate.
2. I love to practice yoga.
3. I love singing to my dog because I don't have a voice and she can't tell me.
4. I love to cook, especially sauces, soups, and things that make the house smell good.
5. I love, love, love (I hope that doesn't count as three) going to the beach any time of the year.
6. I love to be in love.
7. I love to create *anything*.
8. I love to learn and teach new things.
9. I love to be with people.
10. I love to juice-fast and be in silence.

Now it's your turn. Do you love to dance? Take walks? Go to the movies? Be with your family? Whatever it is you love to do, write it down on a piece of paper, numbering from one through ten. The items on your love list don't need to be in any particular order (#1 doesn't have to be your greatest love). The important thing is to write them down. If you have more than ten, that's okay too! If you can't think of ten things right away, don't pressure yourself. Just relax and let yourself meditate on the idea for a while. When I first sat down to write my list, the very first thing I said to myself was, "I don't think I have ten things." It didn't take very long to discover how much I was underestimating myself.

Once you have completed your list, pause for a moment and think about how many of these things you have actually done in the past month, the past six months, and the past year of your life. Most people I meet are doing one or two of the things on their list, and many aren't doing *any*. That is very scary to me. It's scary because if you are only doing one or two or none of the things on your list, your life is very out of balance. If you have lost the connection to the joy in your life, and you're not doing what you love, then your life has become toxic. It's that simple.

Most people get very awakened by this list. They see that over the years they have abandoned the loves of their life, and that today they are nowhere near the vast majority of things they truly love to do. Maybe you have excellent explanations and justifications for each, but the point is that you are still cheating yourself of a rich, full life. I am not telling you this to get you angry or depressed. I am telling you this to help you come awake and come alive. That is why the first thing you need to do right now is to fold up your love list and place it on your altar. By placing your love list on the altar, you are releasing it to your higher power, symbolically asking your higher power to help you reconnect to the love in your life.

FINDING YOUR GUIDE: IF YOU'RE FEELING LOST, YOU NEED A MAP

One of the basic tools you will use to help you make sense of your life story and assist you on your journey of transformation is what I call "life maps." Life maps are a travel aid to carry with you through the fast; they are a way of helping you heal the past. Drawing these maps will make your life history more concrete and real, while opening doors to the future.

The first map I want you to think about is a map of the past. This map will outline the basic themes of your life and give you important clues to where your energy and spirit may be held prisoner. It will help you reflect on joys and disappointments, victory and defeat, left turns, right turns, U-turns, and dead ends, and it will also help you decide how and where you wish to travel in the future. Where have you been, how did you get there, and why did you go? What made you leave or not leave. Where did you have the best time? The worst time? Where are your memories strongest? Where are they weakest? Where are they missing? What was your speed when you traveled down these roads? What were you using for fuel? How much old luggage is still with you today? Your life map of the past will address all these questions.

After this map has been completed, I'm going to ask you to think about a second life map, one that focuses on the present as well as your goals for the future. This map will be a map of hope and inspiration; you can use it to create new dreams and to turn old dreams into practical visions. Life maps give insight, inspiration, and hope, but they should also be fun. So be playful and joyful as you reflect on the past and look to the future. And try to be daring as well. Remember that the 3-Day Detox is about transformation. This is a time for you to be expansive and courageous, and to experience your own creativity and power.

Don't rush; I recommend working on your maps over a period of several days. This will give you a chance to reflect on the questions I'll be asking, and it will help you enhance your maps with important details.

EXERCISE: LIFE MAPS

You will need several notebook-sized sheets of lined paper, and two pencils (with eraser tips). To do this exercise, it is best to be sitting on the floor within your sacred space with all of your materials spread out around you. If this makes you feel like you are back in kindergarten, that's a sure sign that you are doing it right.

If you look back on your life, when would you say that your life as an adult first started? Was it when you graduated from high school? Was it when you dropped out? Was it when you graduated college? Was it when you got your first job? Was it when you lost a parent? Was it when you got married? When you had your first child? Whatever your answer is, write this down. Imagine that someone asked you to create a game called "My Adult Life." What would that game board look like? Would it be a wild maze? A straight line? A series of dizzying circles? Now is your chance to find out.

Begin by taking a piece of the lined notebook paper and dividing it into three columns. At the top of the first column write: "Event." At the top of the second column write: "Reason." At the top of the third column, write: "Impact." In the first column, list all of the things you consider significant events in your adult life: relationship events, job events, family events, moves, health crises, etc., etc. Don't rack your brain to remember things, just write down the things that are most memorable, and that come to mind most quickly.

Now look at each event and think about it for a few moments. Was it an accident? Was it something you chose? Was it something you worked hard for? Was it something you still don't understand? Write a *brief* explanation (four to five words, maximum) for each event in the column labeled Reason. For example, you might write: "I wanted it" or "I was in love" or "I had no choice" or "I pushed too hard" or "I didn't know any better" or "Shit happens." Once again, do not rack your brain. Do not let yourself dwell on or obsess over your answers. Trust your instincts to know that the first response that comes to mind is sufficient. If you can't think of a response quickly, leave it blank.

When you have completed the Reason column, consider each event one last time. Was it a positive event? . . . a negative event? . . . a turning point? On the board game of your adult life, did this event move you ahead? . . . set you back? . . . send you in the wrong direction? . . . make you lose your turn? Write down your answers, keeping them brief (four or five words for each is plenty), in the column labeled Impact. Don't think too hard about your answers and don't get lost in them. The first few words that come to mind are the ones you want to write down. You want to get reacquainted with your past; you don't want to get stuck in it. Creating a map of your past gives you a way to contain it, make sense of it, and ultimately, to discard the parts of it that have been a burden to you. Don't invest too much of your precious emotional energy in things that have already happened—you want to save that energy for building your new future.

Most of us have struggled very hard to get where we are today, even if it's not exactly where we want to be. I don't want to make light of your history, but you should keep your sense of humor and have fun here. This life map is about making peace with the past and letting go so you can move on with your life. If you can't be playful with this map, skip it for now and move on to the second map. You might find it easier to return to once you have created your map for the future.

WISH LIST FOR THE FUTURE

You are about to create a wish list, so take a few moments and give this some serious thought. What do you want to be doing with your life that you aren't doing right now? Think about *everything* from short-term needs to long-term goals. Do you wish you could travel more? Do you wish you could exercise more? Do you wish you could eat in a more healthful way? Do you wish you could lose ten pounds? Do you wish you could find a loving partner? Do you wish you could communicate more with your mate? Do you wish you could leave the relationship you are in? Do you wish you could spend more time with your children? Do you wish you could move? Do you wish you could find a better job? Do you wish you could have tons of money? Do you wish you could save more money? Do you wish you could have a beach house? Do you wish you could fly a plane? Do you wish the car from Publisher's Clearing House would come to your house today? Do you wish you could sing like Barbra Streisand for an hour? Do you wish you could get a dog? Do you wish you could get rid of your anxiety? Do you wish you could quit smoking? Do you wish you could go back to college? Do you wish you could go to more concerts? Do you wish you had roses growing in your yard? Do you wish you could sleep for fifteen more minutes each morning?

Maybe it's an old dream that you are still holding on to, or maybe it's a new dream that has become important to you. Whatever it is, big or small, terribly modest or totally ambitious, write it down on a sheet of your lined paper. Make as long a list as you want. This is the time to let yourself go on a "vision quest"—the deepest quest for who you want to be and what you want to have in your life. Don't hold back *anything*, even if it's something you think might be totally impossible. This is not the time to make that decision; this is the time to be open, to dream, to hope, and to plan. If there was a genie in your life who could grant your wishes, what would these wishes be. This is the time to get inspired by magic. At any time, this wish could come true.

THE SKY'S THE LIMIT—YOUR SPECIAL WISH LIST

Take a good look at all of the items you have placed on your list. Choose *three* of these items—only three, for now—and bring these three wishes to your altar. And open them up to possibility in your life. Don't plan on how this dream could happen. You never know how magic happens. Just leave them on your altar. The most essential thing right now is to stay positive, open, and inspired. This is not the time to think about what could go wrong, what could get in the way, or what has stopped you in the past. This is not the time to doubt or question yourself or your wishes. Instead break down all the limitations that have been placed inside you and access your personal genie. This is a time to explore new possibility and new power.

USING A JOURNAL TO WRITE A NEW LIFE STORY

Remember that this program is about a lot more than giving up solid food for a few days; it's about reflection, growth, healing, and caring. It is immensely valuable to record your thoughts, feelings, fears, doubts, questions, answers, highs, lows, insights, and revelations as you proceed. Journal-writing is essential. Because it helps you remember what you are learning, it helps you activate change. Keeping a journal will solidify your lessons, clarify your goals, calm your fears, expand your self-understanding, strengthen your commitment. This is why I tell everyone who fasts that if you want to feel the power of this process, be absolutely sure to "get it in writing."

Right now—today or tomorrow if at all possible—you need to purchase a notebook or journal and dedicate it to your new journey. You may even want to write in big, beautiful letters on the cover: *My Journey*. (If you're feeling really courageous, you might prefer to write *My Transformation* or *My New Life*.) You may already have a special journal or daily diary but I still recommend that you get a new book exclusively for this venture. The 3-Day Detox is a change of life, and it needs to be honored accordingly in a journal that is brand new and special.

As you read through the three-day program, you will see that I suggest setting aside time every day, both during the prefast and the fast, for your journal-writing. Try to write two or three times each day—or even more if you have the desire. That may sound like a lot of writing, but you're going to have a lot of important things to write about. Right now you may be thinking, "If something really important happens, I'm sure I'll remember it." Too often that isn't the case, especially because so much that is important will be happening in such a very short period of time. If you went on the travel adventure of a lifetime without a camera, you would always have regrets. You may not be getting on a plane or a boat, but this *is* the adventure of a lifetime and you should record it as thoroughly as possible.

Since your fast is a private, self-nurturing ritual—an experience that is yours and yours alone, your journal-writing should be equally private and self-nurturing. Your journal should be a place where you feel alive and free; this is a place where you can feel creative and playful. Draw in it, or color with your crayons or markers. Write about your dreams. Write poetry or prose or songs. Don't be nervous about your creativity, and don't be afraid to have some fun.

I think of the journal as the ultimate scrapbook of metamorphosis—a wonderful place not only to record your experience, but also to save "memorabilia" from your three-day journey. You can press flowers or leaves you collect on your walks. You can collect shells from the beach or stones from the countryside and glue them into your book. You can save the seeds from the fruits and vegetables you'll be juicing. You can record special recipes you think of as you are creating your daily juices. *Anything* that reminds you of this special time can find a caring home within your journal, and that includes the tears from a healing cry.

During the fast, your journal is your mirror—the closest thing you have to yourself that fully reflects who you are. Regardless of what you write, it is always poignant because of what it reflects in you. Your journal is also your container—a place to hold all the ideas you have been carrying in your head, the feelings you've been carrying in your body, and the many new thoughts and feelings that "come up" and need to "get out" during the three days of fasting. And a journal is great to look back on for support, for grounding, and for future inspiration.

For a lot of people, the journal becomes a real buddy during the fast. They take it with them everywhere they go. This close relationship often continues long after the fast is over. If you choose to make fasting a more regular practice in your life, your journal will help you recognize how much you are growing and changing with each fast. You will see how you have come to master challenges that once seemed so difficult and stressful, and your progress will inspire you to set even more new goals.

Keeping a journal is not going to be easy for everybody. So much is leaving you, so much is opening, and so much is being revealed that you may not want to add to your vulnerability by writing about this sensitive process. When I first started keeping a journal I was so self-conscious that I had to make believe I was writing letters to someone else. Over time I got more comfortable, as you will too. I also know that you'll be so glad you struggled through it!

Please remember this: The journal should never be a source of anxiety or stress. It doesn't matter if you're a skilled writer, or a total novice. It doesn't matter if you've kept diaries all your life or if you've never written in a journal before. What you want is a record of what you are shedding and what you are learning—what is going off and what is going on. So be kind to yourself, and let your thoughts, and your pen, flow as freely as possible.

To make my journal-writing feel even more special and sacred, I bought a special pen four years ago that I use only when writing in my journal. Knowing that I am using my journal pen makes the writing process feel even more magical. I recommend it to anyone who is willing to make the small investment. Art supply stores and stationery stores tend to have a large selection of beautiful pens, and they are also some of the best places to find beautiful journals too.

Begin your journal with something very simple. At the top of the first page, write today's date. Underneath the date, write the words: "My Love List." Now copy the list you created into your journal. A journal should begin with inspiration, hope, and love. Your love list will give you all of those, and much more.

Questions, Questions, Questions

Melinda says she can't wait to reap the benefits of the 3-Day Detox program. She says she is ready for cleansing. She says she is ready for healing. Most of all, she says she is ready for change. But Melinda also says that she is not ready to fast. Not yet. Not quite now. Maybe someday soon. But not today, that's for sure. The problem is that Melinda is afraid to fast. Just thinking about the idea of not eating for three days fills her with an incredible sense of dread.

You see, Melinda has tried to go without food before when she was crash-dieting. Two times. Those experiences were horrible. Both times she felt miserable because she didn't know what to do with herself when she wasn't eating. She didn't know what to think about when she wasn't thinking about food. Besides, Melinda felt so deprived during these crash diets that the moment the allotted time was up, she started wolfing down everything in sight. Melinda says that she likes the idea of the Ultimate 3-Day Life Detox, but she has a few questions she needs to have answered before she's ready to give it a try.

Adam would also like to fast, but when he begins to give it serious consideration, all he can think about is his precious morning coffee, the breakfasts he will crave, the late-night snacks he has never gone without, and, most of all, the horrible headaches he feels certain he will have. Okay, maybe he could survive without the breakfasts, maybe he could tough it out without coffee, and maybe he could live without cookies for a few nights, but the headaches . . . just thinking about it has Adam completely paralyzed.

Adam's terror makes a lot of sense if you understand his history. When Adam was a young man, his entire family would follow the Jewish tradition of a one-day fast on Yom Kippur, the most holy day on the Jewish calendar. For Adam, Yom Kippur came to mean only one thing: headaches. By three o'clock in the afternoon, while other members of his family seemed lost in prayer, all Adam could think about was how much his head was hurting. As he got older and older, he started to break his fast earlier and earlier. By the time he was twenty, he had abandoned the practice entirely.

Today, Adam is still afraid of fasting, and he is not alone. Whether it's a fear of giving up coffee and donuts, a fear of feeling crummy, or a fear of what your friends will think, many of us fear the "unknowns" of fasting. Now you need to understand that Adam's fast, though it was only for twenty-four hours, was a very severe fast. Adam was told he could not eat or drink *anything* during the fast. No water. Certainly, no juice! No nothin'. The Yom Kippur tradition of fasting is an extremely important one for those of us who practice it, yet I also know that lots of people might feel awful on a fast like this, even if it is just for one day. While the fast I am offering to you isn't anything like Adam's Yom Kippur fast of twenty-four hours without food, it is still a fast, and that can be pretty scary.

As far as I'm concerned, every fear of fasting is a valid one. That's why it's my job to make most of these unknowns *known*. The more I can demystify the experience of fasting right now, the more you are going to trust me, trust your body, and trust the process. And that brings us to the first question. . . .

IS THERE A RIGHT WAY AND A WRONG WAY TO FAST?

There are all kinds of ways to fast. Believe me, I've tried most of them. Many of the fasting methods that are being advocated are extreme as well as harsh. Everything starts happening too fast. The truth is that if you fast on nothing but water, for example, it can shock all of your systems and make you ill. Physiologically, you start detoxing too quickly, and that can put too much of a burden on your body. Emotionally it can wipe you out because it makes you feel deprived. A harsh fast is not spiritually helpful because it's so overwhelming, you don't know what to think about. In my experience, a water fast can turn into "water torture" very quickly.

Some people say you shouldn't eat or drink *anything* when you fast. That's a really great way to get sick *fast*. Another popular fast is the brown rice fast. This can be good in the deep of winter, when the body needs a little more than just juice. If it's cold outside and your body is in its winter hibernation, but you still want to go on some kind of a fast, you might find that brown rice and broth is very soothing. I do recommend it to a lot of people, but I also think it's too heavy for spring, summer, or even early fall. Besides, rice doesn't give your digestive system a chance to turn off the way juice does, so you're not going to get the same kind of a detox in three days.

Then there are all the exotic fasts you hear about from time to time. Sauerkraut juice concoctions, olive oil flushes, cayenne and chile pepper elixirs . . . I've tried most of them and I have to admit that some are very interesting and some are very powerful. I also need to admit that some are absolutely disgusting, and a few are probably dangerous. My overall feeling is that most of these exotic fasts are just not necessary. The experience of fasting doesn't have to be austere and painful, it can be rich and beautiful while still being powerful and profound. The secret to making it so special is fasting with fresh juices. I didn't have to go to a mountaintop and suffer to cleanse and become healthy. Why should you?

HOW WILL I FEEL WHILE I'M FASTING?

One of the hardest things about detox is all of the funky symptoms that start appearing as your toxins start to exit the body. Every toxin seems to have an "exit signature," its own unpleasant way of saying good-bye to the body that has been such a gracious host. That bag of chocolate chip cookies may taste good going in but don't be surprised if it says good-bye with a rash, some acne, or even a couple of large, ugly pimples. It's not fun, I know. But you are doing an incredible thing for yourself and it's worth it! I think the most important thing is to be prepared, so you are not surprised or frightened if an unpleasant symptom surfaces. Some people will experience none of this. But if you've spent a year in an office with rotten ventilation, eating rich food and wine, figure that you've spent a year on a toxic cruise ship, and expect to have some unpleasant "side effects." For example, you may:

- get itchy
- have bad breath
- perspire more than usual
- get pimples
- have watery eyes
- have a funny taste in your mouth
- get backaches and muscle cramps

You will probably urinate more than usual, and your bowel pattern will change. Your memory may seem a little foggy. Also, watch out for small mood swings. Feelings that are usually under the surface can move forward and you may get a little irritable and cranky.

This is a list of *possible* symptoms, not a profile of the typical individual experience. While any of these things *could* happen, I don't know anybody who has had them *all* happen during a three-day detox. Some people don't have any of them. Obviously, a very complicated process is taking place within your body. Your job is to witness this cleaning out without getting alarmed.

That, as they say, is the bad news. Now let me give you some good news. These symptoms should be an inspiration to you during the fast. Why? Because you *want* to see this happen! These symptoms are proof positive that your body is cleansing itself.

These symptoms shouldn't last very long. Some last only a few hours, some last only a few minutes. None are permanent. And when they pass, you feel great. This is not a setup for the old "why do you keep hitting yourself on the head? Because it feels so good when I stop" joke. Once a symptom passes, you are likely to feel much better than you ever felt before any symptoms began. The other thing is that you probably will only have one symptom at a time. Once it moves on, another one may move in briefly.

There's no need to suffer. Rest or sleep helps many of these symptoms pass. Other symptoms can be minimized or alleviated entirely by drinking more water.

There is one final point I need to make here. Most people who are interested in fasting are already fairly healthy. People like this typically have minimal discomfort during the fast. If you have been doing things that really punish the body for years and years, your first fast could produce more intense versions of some of the above symptoms. Some alternative healing professionals call these reactions a "healing event." It sounds great, and it is great, because a healing event is a sure sign that you have been very toxic; but it is also very intense, and possibly even a little bit frightening. Being prepared will make this less frightening. I need to state very clearly that if, for any reason you start to feel really ill, or you become too scared to continue your fast, *Do Not Continue Your Fast*. If you have *any*, and I mean *any* reason to believe that you will have a difficult time dealing with a three-day juice fast, it is essential that you get clearance from your doctor. Even if you do not complete all three days of fasting, it is very important to carefully follow the guidelines for breaking the fast as presented in Chapter 13.

WHAT ARE *MY* CHANCES OF GETTING SYMPTOMS?

It depends on your body type; it depends on your diet; it depends on your general health; and it depends on your history with toxic substances—foods, drugs, environmental toxins, etc. Most important, it depends on your attitude.

There are a few things you can pretty much count on. If you have been eating lots of red meat or drinking too much alcohol, you may have some small discomfort; if you are accustomed to drinking a lot of coffee, you're probably going to get a headache the first day of the fast; if you're a sugar junkie, you might get a headache or feel cranky.

Anything that has been trapped inside of your body will be heading for the exits during your detox. More than anyone, you are the expert on what has gone into your body over the years that could be hiding somewhere in storage. That means that, more than anyone, you have the best sense of what might be ready to come out. I'm not saying this to scare you, only to prepare you. Fasting does make you face your past, and that can be unpleasant for those of us who have tried our best to forget about all of the things that we have put in our bodies. That's why you need to think about this: Cleaning out the past—whatever that may be—is your ticket to a new and different future.

ANY OTHER "SURPRISES" I NEED TO KNOW ABOUT?

During this deep cleansing, you are also peeling away your history. You can find yourself "time traveling" through all kinds of things from your past: old emotions, old dreams, old memories, old behaviors. . . . Sometimes you can sense what it is that you are revisiting, yet other times you could feel confused. Particularly since these old pieces of you may come out in a jumble. It's an absolutely fascinating process, but one you should be prepared for.

Part of this retracing process is something I call a "craving regression." When your body is retracing, you can experience powerful cravings for many of the different foods you ate throughout your life, particularly the comfort foods—triple pepperoni pizzas you had in college, the Christmas ham you had when you were fifteen, oatmeal you had when you were six, banana pudding you adored when you were two. . . . This can feel very weird, but it's also a lot of fun. It's a trip down memory lane that makes you feel like you're a little kid again. And in a way, you are. You are going deep into your body to pull out all of the bad stuff you've been storing since you were a little kid; it shouldn't be surprising that you're going to pull up all kinds of childhood "food memories" along with it. Is it hard to imagine that our cells have this kind of memory? There was a time in my life when it was hard for me to imagine too. Recently I was watching one of the morning news programs, and they showed a clip of a little girl, she couldn't have been more than eight or nine, who was recovering from a serious illness. She had received a bone marrow transplant from a man whom she was meeting for the first time, and she had an incredible question to ask him. In the news clip, she looked at him and asked, "Do you like Chinese food?" "Yes," he answered, "why?" "I thought so," she said, "because ever since I got your bone marrow, I keep thinking about Chinese food."

For me this story is just a confirmation of what I've already experienced. I still remember the craving regressions I had the first time I ever fasted. I had such a taste for the corn niblets and fried chicken my mother made for me when I was twelve. I would actually taste these things on my tongue and think, "What is going on here?" I was not well prepared for this experience, which is one of the reasons I want to make sure that you are.

Retracing is much more profound on a long fast than on a relatively short fast like the 3-Day Detox. And you may not even have a craving regression on your three-day fast. If it does happen to you, you need to know that you're not going nuts and you're probably not pregnant. You are merely retracing your food history.

WILL I BE HUNGRY THE ENTIRE TIME?

People get so panicky about leaving food behind that this is all they can think about when they think about fasting. Hunger is such a loaded emotional experience for most of us. It brings up issues with love, loss, abandonment, denial, deprivation. No wonder it is so terrifying. That's why I need to say something right now to put your mind more at ease: *You are not breaking up with food, you are just taking separate vacations.* This fast is only three days, it is not forever. After that, you and your favorite foods will be reunited, and the relationship will be a much healthier one. So take a few deep breaths and relax.

Now here's the surprise: Fasting is not synonymous with hunger, and the secret is in the juice. Your body will be getting so many nutrients and so much nourishment from the juices and broths you will be drinking that you will probably stop thinking about food. I need to say that again: *You will probably stop thinking about food!* Granted, this does not happen to everyone. If you're used to stuffing yourself silly, you're more likely to struggle. But more often than not, this is the typical experience of someone who goes on a juice fast. This is one of the amazing truths of juice-fasting.

One of the biggest problems I have with the people who go on this juice fast is the exact opposite of what you would ever expect: they lose their appetite after the first day, and don't always drink *enough* juice. They actually start forgetting to drink their juice. Can you imagine actually skipping meals by accident during a fast? Sounds crazy, I know, but it happens to people so often that I need to warn you that it could happen to you.

As you look through the contents of Days 1, 2, and 3, you will notice that I have clearly stated very specific *minimums* for every meal of the fast. *Minimums.* You really can drink as much as you want on this fast, but it's very important to at least drink the minimum at every single meal. And: *Skipping meals is a no-no.*

Right now, you may find this very amusing. Right now, you may be absolutely convinced that you'll be obsessing about food every single moment of your three waking fast days, and dreaming about food every night. Maybe that's true, but it's far more likely that you will be both surprised and delighted by the shift inside of you that is about to take place.

CAN I DRINK COFFEE OR ALCOHOL?

How many ways can I say no? ABSOLUTELY NO, NO, NO!!!! Alcohol and coffee—even decaffeinated coffee—bring way too many toxins *into* the system. You want toxins to be flowing in only one direction during your fast: *Out*.

Teas with caffeine and decaffeinated teas aren't any better. Herbal teas, on the other hand, are a very different story. I encourage people to sip herbal teas throughout the day during all three fasting days.

CAN I SMOKE?

PLEASE don't. Smoking is toxic, period. Try not to smoke, or try to give up smoking during the fasting process. Start cutting back before the fast so you don't have to go cold turkey. I know how hard it is to even *think* about not smoking for a few days. It was a very hard addiction for me to give up. Fasting and smoking (cigarettes, cigars, or pipes) just don't mix. Now the good news: Many people lose all interest in smoking once they have completed their first three-day detox.

CAN I FILL UP BEFORE I FAST?

Some people want to eat everything in sight before they start their fast. They think this will make it easier to give up food for a few days. The fact is it makes it much harder. Stuffing yourself silly before a fast stretches the stomach, increasing your craving for food during the fast. It also postpones the cleansing and detoxification of your system by keeping your digestive system active and cranking at its full power. You want to give your system a rest. The last thing you need is to be spending your three days of fasting digesting your "last supper."

SHOULD I TAKE SUPPLEMENTS?

I'm a big believer in taking vitamin and herbal supplements, but not during a fast. Vitamin supplements should always be taken with solid food to assist in their proper breakdown and absorption. Without solid food in your diet, vitamin pills will put extra strain on the liver, and on your kidneys too. This is never healthy, but during a fast it is particularly unhealthy. Taking vitamins also interferes with the detox process. The primary purpose of this fast is to make your digestion stop so that your body can go after what it doesn't need. Vitamins have to be digested, and that keeps the system going. If you don't give your body a complete rest from digestion, you won't fully activate your detox.

IF I DON'T TAKE SUPPLEMENTS, WILL MY BODY BE GETTING EVERYTHING IT NEEDS?

It's only three days. Your body will be getting *more* than it needs. The juice and broth recipes in this program have been designed very carefully to ensure that you are getting all of the vitamins, minerals, and trace elements you require, and visible proof will come very quickly. Before three days have passed your skin and hair will be glowing with a new sense of vitality and your eyes will be more clear, more alive, and more vibrant. If you have food allergies, those symptoms may even disappear, which is a wonderful and often unexpected bonus. Most important, you are going to *feel* more alive—perhaps more alive than you could ever remember. To me, that is the ultimate proof that your body is being well fed.

WHAT ABOUT MEDICATION?

Fasting does not mix very well with many medications. IF YOU ARE TAKING MEDICATION, IT IS IMPORTANT TO DISCUSS YOUR INTENTION TO DETOX WITH YOUR PRESCRIBING PHYSICIAN.

Once you are fasting, you do not want to use medicine to treat your fasting/detox symptoms. This means no aspirin, Tylenol, or other painkillers; no pink bismuth drinks or white minty drinks for stomach upset (if you have digestive upsets of any kind, discuss fasting with your doctor before you begin); no sleeping aids for restlessness; etc. If you are a regular consumer of these things, or a self-medicator, I would like it if you could stop your intake of these chemicals during the fast. This is the kind of stuff you want to get *out* of your system during the fast, not put *in*.

WILL I HAVE ANY ENERGY?

So many people think that during the fasting experience they will look like Gandhi in the last years of his life. All they can envision is a feeble body with a cane and loincloth, weighed down by the burdens of the universe. If you don't have a cane, loincloth, or feeble body right now, you aren't going to get that way from the fast I recommend. Your energy should actually *increase* as each day goes by. That's part of what makes the experience so powerful. You get stronger, you get healthier, and you look the part.

WHAT'S THE WORST THING THAT CAN HAPPEN?

Some people, particularly people who have never fasted before, start thinking about worst-case scenarios before they start fasting. They wonder about things like, "What if I don't like the way I feel?" "What if I get scared?" "What if I'm miserable?" "What if I can't go on?" "What if I absolutely positively *have* to eat?" I have one very simple answer for all of these questions: *You eat*.

If, for any reason, you don't want to continue your fast, then *don't* continue your fast. It's that simple. There's nothing wrong with stopping. And there's nothing unhealthy about stopping before the three days are over, provided you break your fast slowly and carefully, as described in Chapter 13.

You are doing this for yourself, and, as far as I'm concerned, you don't have anything to prove to *anyone*. Stopping the fast before the three days are over doesn't make you a failure and it doesn't make you a bad person. You may decide to try again next year, or next month, or even next week. You may decide that one or two days was enough for you this time around. Yes, this program has been designed to last three full days, and it is my hope that you take full advantage of that design. But that doesn't mean you won't experience any of the program's benefits if, for whatever reason, you do not complete all three days of fasting. The most important thing is that you always know that you can quit whenever you want to quit.

CAN I FAST TO LOSE WEIGHT?

The fast I advocate is not a weight-loss program. This is a cleansing program, not a diet. I need to say that again, and I want you to say it with me: *This is a cleansing program, not a diet.* A three-day fast is a great introduction to a new way of being with food, and yes, if you are overweight, you will probably lose *some* weight. That's great. But the fast is not a diet. It can help drop you to your "natural" weight, but if your natural weight is only one pound less than you weigh now, you are not going to drop any further. This can be frustrating to anyone who is desperate to lose five pounds.

I just worked with a woman who was absolutely miserable because she couldn't lose any weight. She exercised every morning, played tennis every afternoon, swam after tennis, and then *maybe* had a piece of fruit and half a dry, toasted bagel. She was in incredible shape, but in her mind, she *had* to lose five pounds to be at her perfect weight. She was certain that fasting would bring her weight down. It didn't. She did lose three pounds during her fast, which got her very excited, but two pounds came back within a few days, and that made her miserable. I told her that her body needed the weight. She told me she felt like a failure. Despite the fact that I discouraged this woman from having any kind of expectations concerning weight loss, she was so unhappy that she was unable to appreciate the many wonderful things that fasting *was* bringing her.

This fast lasts only three days. Three days is all you need, and three days is all I recommend. If you are searching for a diet, you need to find a way of eating that you can practice for longer periods of time, if not *all* the time. Fasting, in my opinion, is just not the answer. Besides, I don't believe in diets; I believe in changing your lifestyle. Weight loss is a challenge to many men and women, and there are a million programs out there designed to help people eat right and/or exercise more. But cleaning out is another story. We are talking about doing a different level of work here. This is an emotional, spiritual, *and* physical program.

Now here's a surprise I need to prepare you for: on the first day or two of the fast, your body might bloat up from the toxins and you could actually *gain* a little weight. This is particularly true for many women who have a history of dieting and deprivation. What happens is that the thought of going on a fast actually scares the body. The body retaliates by instantly saying "not again," and you start to put on weight. People ask me, "How can I be gaining weight during a fast?" If this happens to you, understand that your body is still frightened by your dieting history and it doesn't trust this new process yet. But it will. Once it starts feeling good from emptying out, something will let go and the weight you gained will drop off.

You should also know that on this fast, you may not lose any weight until several days *after* your fast is over. The juices you will be drinking stop your body from losing those initial few pounds of water weight that come off in the beginning of most diets (and go back on shortly thereafter). That can be disappointing to people who are used to losing five quick pounds whenever they start any kind of a controlled food regimen. This is why I ask everyone *PLEASE, do not* step on a scale during your fast. Do not weigh yourself. Don't even think about it. You don't want to get confused, you don't want to become obsessed, and you don't want to sabotage the process. By staying off the scale, you will be doing yourself a great favor, and keeping your focus off the issue of weight as much as possible.

I'm going to say it one last time: *This fast is not a diet*, and should never be used for dieting purposes. Fasting is an extraordinary way to learn about your body's relationship to food, and how you can change that relationship. I find that within one year of their first fast, most people have completely changed the way they eat. A three-day cleansing fast will help your body get rid of the memory of all that sugar, wheat, caffeine, and processed food. Then when you reintroduce these and other foods back into your diet, typically your reactions will make you aware of your specific sensitivities. Fasting teaches you about the foods that make you anxious, the foods that make you gaseous, the foods that make you sad, the foods that slow you down, and the foods that make you sick. Fasting teaches you about all the foods you can live very happily without, and all the foods you can live very happily with. But it is a teacher. It is not a lifestyle.

WILL FASTING HAVE ANY EFFECT ON HOW I LOOK?

Yes, all that fresh juice will make your skin glow. It will make your eyes bright and your hair shine. And, oh yes, one of the best things to happen from a three-day fast: Your stomach will look and feel flatter and less bloated. That's because you haven't been eating pasta, bread, or any other wheat products.

When you finish with your fast, people will probably comment that you have never looked better.

IF I AM SICK, CAN FASTING MAKE ME WELL?

The 3-Day Energy Fast does not treat, diagnose, or claim to cure any disease or condition. The 3-Day Energy Fast is also not intended to be a substitute for any drug or medical procedure. If you are sick, if you have recently been sick, or if you have any chronic medical condition, discuss your interest in fasting with your physician before you proceed with this or any other fasting program. While it is true that fasting promotes health, fasting is also a challenge to the body. Sure, I have seen, heard, and read about many fasting cures, I have also seen, heard, and read about health problems that are exacerbated by fasting. A lot of fasting experts see fasting as the answer for everything, but I cannot support that position. And whether you are sick or well, you should *always* check with your doctor or practitioner before going on *any* fast, including this one.

CAN I WORK WHILE I FAST?

Yes, but you would be kinder to yourself if you choose not to. If this is your first fast, I recommend that you do it on a three-day weekend, or during any three consecutive vacation days. You really want to treat these three days as though you were on a retreat, and your office is the last place you need to go during a retreat. I realize, however, that there are a lot of people who just can't take three days off from work. Can they still do the program? Absolutely.

I have detoxed on the job when I had no other choice. I have even detoxed on the road, when I was traveling for my job. It's not the best way to do it, but it's not impossible either. I do, however, have a few suggestions for those of you who can't stay home, and here is the first and most important one: I think it is very important that you at least *begin* the fast on a day you don't have to work. If you can, fast on Saturday and Sunday and work on Monday, the third day, when you should get a natural boost in energy from the detox process.

You are going to need Day 1—the first day of the fast—to get acquainted with all of the changes you'll be introducing. If you must go back to work on Day 2 or Day 3, then go back to work. You can prepare all of the juices and drinks you'll need each morning of the fast before you go to work, so you won't have to carry a twenty-pound juicer and a blender to your office every day (although you could if you wanted to!). And you can make a few other adjustments to accommodate your special juice regimen. You can, for example, get a couple of thermos bottles to keep your juice cool and your broth warm. You can even make some of your fruit drinks in the evening and freeze them. The next day, let them thaw at the office until they are ready to drink (in the summer, you might enjoy drinking them as icy slushes).

Some people use their jobs as an excuse *not* to fast. They tell me things like, "I don't have a refrigerator," "I don't have time for any meals, not even for juice," "What if I have to schedule a last-minute lunch appointment?" These are all ways of avoiding fasting. The fact is that if you have the intention to fast, you can do it. After all, it's *only* three days. Many people drink springwater all day, and they bring their bottles to work. People who feel they need to smoke cigarettes find a way to do it in the office, don't they? How about you? If you like coffee and snacks, you figure out the schedule of the snack service . . . don't you? If you can accommodate your other needs, you can accommodate this program. There is nothing about this juice fast that you cannot adapt to your workplace *if you have the desire*.

CAN I STILL WORK OUT WHILE I FAST?

Do you need to run 10k just to start the day? Is it hard to imagine 108 hours away from your NordicTrack? Have you never missed an evening at the gym? Then you're probably not going to like what I am about to say: *Rigorous* exercise is another fasting no-no.

You may be resting your feet a lot during the fast, but the rest of your body is going to be working incredibly hard cleansing itself. You don't want to add to that load and put an unhealthy strain on your system with excessive exercise. Your body needs to stay focused on the major task it will be doing during these three days: Detox. The last thing you need is to be diverting your vital energy into a fight-to-the-death tennis game or bun-burning workout. That's why the only exercises I recommend are gentle exercises like yoga, walking, swimming, biking, and breath work that support and enhance the fast. These exercises, which are *very important*, will greatly enhance the detox process. For three days, they are all the exercise you will need.

WHAT ABOUT MY FAMILY?

Sometimes partners, family members, or friends want to get into the act. They may, for example, offer to give up some of their meals to drink juice with you. That can feel very loving and supportive if it is something you are open to (but *only* if it is something you are open to). But what if they want to follow the entire program?

The 3-Day Energy Fast was designed to be a very private, self-nurturing ritual, and it is important for you to have a lot of time alone. It is in this alone time that the program is often most powerful, and it would be a shame to deprive yourself of such a unique opportunity. I also need to say that if you are craving silence and separateness right now, it can be distracting and frustrating to have other people around you constantly, even if these other people are fasting.

Now, at the risk of contradicting myself, I must also tell you that there have been times that I have done this program with one or two friends and the experience was absolutely beautiful. If you should choose to follow this program with a partner, the most important thing to remember is that everybody's experience is different, and, more than anything, you need to pay attention to your own experience. Caretaking another person, or losing your focus, will leave you shortchanged. When you are fasting, you always want to maintain your separateness, even if you are in the presence of another.

IS THE PROGRAM ALWAYS THE SAME?

Absolutely not. Your juice fast can be season-friendly. The fruits and vegetables your market carries change from spring to summer to fall, and so do the juices in your fast to accommodate those changes. A healthy program needs to be in harmony with nature, not working against it.

These days, it seems as if you can get any kind of fruit or vegetable any time of the year, no matter where you live—you can find honeydew melon in February in New Jersey and asparagus in January in Connecticut. This may be true, but it doesn't mean it is the best thing for you. People used to tell me never to eat anything that is growing more than three hundred miles from where you live. I love that thought, but it's not always practical. For example, those asparagus are coming from California—definitely beyond the limit for a resident of the East Coast. I also would add something else: You don't want to eat any scary "all-season" produce that was grown in a laboratory or produce factory. You don't need to live your life this way. That is a personal choice, and sometimes we need to trade convenience for perfect food choices, but these are very important rules to hold on to during the fast.

Some of the drinks in this three-day program, such as the Morning Drink, are exactly the same year-round. Other drinks can be selected according to the season you are in, the climate you are in, and, of course, the availability of produce. As you read through the fast, you will see that I have always included a number of options in your juice menu to accommodate seasonal differences and regional differences.

The most important rule of thumb I can offer you is really a single word: balance. If, for example, you drank nothing but mango and raspberry juice for three days, you'd get too high from the sugar and get headaches *no matter where you live.* I always recommend diluting your juices with springwater. So keep this in mind and try to make sensible choices.

ARE THERE BAD TIMES TO FAST?

Fasting depends on your needs, it depends on the circumstances in your life, it depends on your schedule, it depends on your health, and it depends on your frame of mind. A general rule of thumb is not to fast when you have too much stress in your life. If you are changing jobs, moving, in the middle of the worst part of a divorce or breakup, or dealing with the illness or loss of a family member or close friend, you don't want to be fasting.

There are other bad times. During the holiday season, when you know you are going to be surrounded by tempting foods for weeks; if you have a calendar packed full of dinner engagements that you have to honor; if you are under extraordinary pressure from work deadlines; if, *for whatever reason*, you're not sure that you have three full days right now to devote yourself to this program. If you can't fast right now, the best thing to do is to accept your inability to make healthier choices right now. Make a plan and a promise to yourself to fast as soon as your circumstances shift. I'd even put it in writing so you know it's something you can trust.

WHAT ARE SOME GOOD TIMES TO FAST?

A fast is a great way to help you make a transition from one state of mind to another. Fasting is basically an intuitive process. Your body tells you when it wants to fast, especially if you have already had the fasting experience. So if your breakup or your divorce is over and you want a little help in moving on, this juice fast is the perfect vehicle. Some people also like to fast right before they start a new job, after the holidays, or after a vacation. This program of fasting, meditation, and ritual especially lends itself to the decision-making process. This is like a perfect three-day retreat to help you make up your mind about anything important.

WHEN CAN I START FASTING?

If you are reading this book for the first time, you may want to start the 3-Day Detox right away. It's great when people are that enthusiastic, and it is certainly something I don't want to discourage. Now that you have read a little bit more about this program and what it entails, stop for a moment and ask yourself: Is now a good time for me to be doing this? I like to think of this fast as a "weekend for the body"—I also like to think that you know better than anyone when you need that weekend. So ask yourself the question and listen carefully to the answer that is inside of you.

If the answer you hear first and loudest is No, I urge you to respect that answer and wait for a better opportunity. Sometimes, waiting even one week can mean the difference between a successful fast and disappointment. If, on the other hand, the answer you hear is a resounding Yes!, then it's time to turn the page and start to prepare.

PART TWO

PREPARING FOR A MIRACLE

People always ask me exactly what it is that they will be doing during the 3-Day Energy Fast. What will they be doing with their time, what will they be doing with their thoughts, what will they be doing with their cravings, and what will they be doing with the demands of the outside world? During these three precious days, you and I will be working together to create something new—*a new you*. This new you is going to shed old habits and old fantasies, as well as old thought patterns and old ways of relating to food.

I'm going to ask you to give up a whole bunch of things, and I'm going to ask you to do a whole bunch of new things. Some of these things may seem very simple, but try to surrender some of the modern-day cynicism we all carry and see what happens.

If you think this fast is just about giving up solid food, you have a far too limited view. Think larger, think deeper. Fasting is about the journey from one place in your life to another. During these three days, everything could seem more precious, more fragile—a little foggier or a lot clearer. You will certainly be living in the moment, which is the only time we really have.

Establishing Some New Rituals

One of the best things about these three days is that you are going to be able to establish new, and better, rituals for living. With energy and love, our daily rituals can rise above mere habit and enter into the domain of the sacred. I believe that each of us is here on this planet for a purpose. Perhaps you know what your purpose is, or perhaps you're only now beginning to look for your own unique sacred purpose. Whatever your journey, I know that discipline and these new rituals will help you find your way to your spiritual center.

Instead of just "doing stuff" with little thought or focus, ritual brings a sense of purpose and purposefulness to your actions. Ritual heightens your awareness, your sensitivity, and your receptivity. Whether it's a way of eating, a way of resting, a way of cleansing, a way of meditating, or even a way of making juice, approaching these acts as ritual elevates them from the ordinary to the sacred, giving your life a feeling of purpose.

These fasting days are presenting you with an opportunity to create powerful and meaningful new rituals that will not only enhance and support your fast, but also have a place in your day-to-day life long after the fast has ended.

SKIN-BRUSHING

Every morning and every evening of the fast, I'm going to ask you to spend at least five minutes focusing on your body in a special way. I want you to establish the ritual of dry brushing your skin with a comfortable, natural fiber body brush. (See pages 127–28 for guidance on skin-brushing.) Since your skin is, technically, your largest organ of elimination, it deserves some extra attention. You want to do everything you can to keep your surface blood circulation strong, keep your pores open and clean, and keep your skin feeling alive. This means you want to be clearing away dead skin cells, as well as toxins that are making their way to the skin surface. And that's where skin-brushing comes in.

Removing dead skin cells and surface toxins with skin-brushing encourages the creation of new cells, while helping your lymphatic system to cleanse and flush itself. Yes, the skin *is* a self-cleaning organ, but it works slowly, and it doesn't always do such a great job. Skin-brushing is like hiring a team of cleaning professionals to do the work. It's much faster, it's super-efficient, and it brings your skin to life in a way you've probably never experienced before. It's like a facial and cell renewal treatment for the skin on your body.

Skin-brushing puts a rosy shine on the skin by stimulating circulation. If you have dry patches or uneven tone, skin-brushing can change that fast. It's off with the old and make room for the new. The newer your cell structure, the newer and more alive you will feel. Deep inside your body, you're using cleansing and revitalizing juices to work their magic, but on the outside surface, skin-brushing is the ticket.

CONSCIOUS BATHING

It's time to relax, let go of your hurried and harried attitude, and see bathing for what it is—a beautiful transforming ritual. I'm sure that many of you gave up baths in favor of showers many years ago. Well, for three days, I'm encouraging you to change your habits and use the bathing ritual. But if you *must* shower, keep the intention of allowing water to soothe and cleanse. Relax and let the water wash over you.

Warm water encourages the pores to open, and that means you are making bigger "pipes" from which the toxins can come pouring out. With all of that toxic material that is finally being freed up from deep inside, you want to do everything you can to insure that it finds its way out. At the same time, you want to be sure to wash away all of the dead cells you've freed up from your skin-brushing. Yes, you could do that with just a shower, but bathing does a better job, and it offers a lot more.

Water is healing. Water therapy is soothing, balancing, calming, protective, and nurturing. It's no accident that water has always been used for baptism, symbolizing a new birth, and a new you. For me, water was my original "elixir." Going to the water has always changed me and it has always cured me. As a child, I spent many, many days at the beach just across the street from where my grandmother lived. I used to stare at the water. I didn't know it then but it was a childhood meditation. Later, when I started going to school, my first school was also right across from the beach. I was the only child who would go to school an hour *early*—especially when I wasn't feeling well—just to go to the beach.

While few of us can get to the beach on a regular basis to feel the healing effects of the water, all of us can spend thirty minutes luxuriating in a beautiful bath. So take the time that you so fully deserve and surrender to the water. Your bath time should be your sacred, private time, and a place for absolute indulgence. Use the time for reflection, and use the water as a mirror for reflecting—a place where you can notice the changes in your skin, your body, and how you feel. Invite the water to enter your pores and carry out all of the things your body no longer wants. Ask it to cleanse you, to free you, and to float you.

In my bathtub I have a pillow and all kinds of bath toys. My toys, all of which I love, include a motorized brush that covers the body with foam, exotic natural sponges, and special lathering soaps. I even have a little floating duck. Sometimes I light candles. Sometimes I play music. And I *always* add special scents to the bathwater. I want you to take the time to do this also because it's going to make you feel terrific.

Many spas are now offering aromatherapy baths as a preferred healing treatment. In the mornings, adding rosemary and basil to the bath will invigorate you. When you go to the store, be certain to buy the oils, not the herbs—you don't want to make soup by mistake. In the evenings, adding scents such as lavender and chamomile, or hops, to your bath will soothe you. A drop of lavender on your bedroom pillow at night will also help the body calm down, and help you sleep.

The most important bath ingredient for opening the pores and encouraging detox is a container of bath salts. People travel thousands of miles to get to spas where they are dunked in salts from the Dead Sea, for example. Once you've done it, you'll see for yourself how calming it can be. Sea salts do a great job of purifying the system. Epsom salts purify too, and they also take away aches and pains.

MEDITATION

Most of us have heard that "prayer is talking to God; meditation is listening." Personally I need to do a lot of listening, and I think most people feel the same way. I need to listen so that I can find the space that comes from my deepest sense of self. If you're raging about your life, you're not listening. If you are obsessing, you're not listening. If you're shopping, you're not listening. Meditation gives you an opportunity to stop and listen to what you need to hear so that you can lead your life in a way that makes you feel happy, healthy, and full.

Meditation is a healing ritual in itself, and a daily dose is an important practice during your days of fasting. Meditation stills the mind and calms the body. When you meditate, you are taking time out from preoccupations, worries, distractions, demands, and other pressures, and creating a quiet space where you can find peace, groundedness, energy, aliveness, and, most important, new answers. In that very special place of quiet, many people make their first connection to a true feeling of spirituality, or reconnect to past spiritual experiences that somehow got lost.

Use Meditation to Get Answers

The two questions I always ask myself are: "What did I come here to learn?" "What did I come here to teach?" These are my questions. Perhaps they're also your questions. Or maybe you have different questions that you want answered for yourself, questions such as: "Should I take this job?" "Should I stay in this relationship?" "Should I have a child?" "Should I move to Colorado?" If you are ready for answers, meditation is the healthiest place to turn for those answers.

Where do your answers come from? Some people feel that the answers to their questions come directly from God. Others feel that they are helped by angels or archangels. Some people believe that they are guided by spirits. Many people pooh-pooh divine intervention. After all, God may be too busy at the moment to attend to every one of your immediate issues. These men and women feel that their answers come directly from their own centers—the wisdom we all carry within ourselves. Whatever you believe or think, I want to assure you that meditation will help you get answers to your questions.

The most important meditations in this book are the daily guided morning meditations included for each day of your fast. These meditations will soothe you, support you, and honor your intention every day of your fasting journey. In addition to preparing you for the day, your guided morning meditation will help you feel relaxed, clear, and cheerful. Over the course of three days, fasting can stir anxiety and stress. A daily ritual of meditation can be one of your most powerful allies, helping you put down any internal rebellions that attempt to disrupt your fast.

The first time I meditated, I expected to have a movie go off in my head; I waited for pictures and sounds. Instead it was complete silence, which is just what I needed. I thought I fell asleep. Some people do fall asleep, and that's perfectly okay. It means your body needs the rest. The most important thing is to keep trying. Reaching nirvana is not the goal here. The only goal is to make it a daily practice—eighteen to twenty minutes a day is ideal.

I love the meditations in this book, but I don't want you to feel restricted by them. If you have your own style of meditation that you are already comfortable with, you should feel free to use that in conjunction with, or as a substitute for, anything offered in this book.

THE RITUAL OF SACRED SILENCE

In this day and age, silence is truly a blessing. Starting a ritual that allows you to find daily periods of silence is an essential way to get connected to the bigger picture. True silence is a spiritual act, and it will help you reach your energy and make your life canvas clear.

I call silence the great leveler. It takes all of our words, the profound ones and the empty ones, mixes them all together, then filters out what we don't need. When you are ready to speak again, your voice will sound calmer, purer, and more balanced. For me, it almost feels as though I'm channeling my own sentences.

Just as juice cleanses the organs and tissues, silence cleanses the psyche by bathing all of the places inside where there is still screaming and tantrums and crying and other painful noise. Silence cradles you, offering a lullaby to the system that is so peaceful and calm. It's like watching a beautiful sunset at the end of the day and that transcendent feeling you get when you let nature wash over you. Your entire spirit feels calmed and soothed.

Make room for yourself by enjoying at least fifteen or twenty minutes of silent time every day that you are fasting. Try building this up by adding ten or fifteen minutes each day. This is not a time to read or write, walk the dog, or do the dishes. It is a time to just sit calmly and be with yourself. This is something we all need to do. Does that sound easy? Well, it isn't. When you first try to be silent, the first thing that happens is that the chatter gets louder and louder in your head. If you ever give yourself several days of silence, you may discover that the chatter continues through Day 1. It's often not until the second or third day before the chatter stops engaging you. For people who struggle with anxiety, getting and staying silent can be one of the greatest challenges of all during the fast. The first time I tried to be silent I couldn't sit still. I actually got on my bicycle and pedaled to my place of business, then wrote out a note to the manager reminding her of something I knew she had forgotten. I felt like the witch in the Wizard of Oz. Even in the silence, my control issues still had control of me. So much has changed in my life since then, and silence has been an important catalyst for that change.

When you close your eyes to get silent and calm the body, the first thing that usually happens is that a "silent movie" starts playing in your head, right in front of your eyes, in a way that you can actually see it. It is very important to let the movie play. This is the story that lives inside you—the story that keeps your life noisy, that makes you chat constantly, that stops you from truly resting, relaxing, and being still.

Some people have a soundtrack to their movie; some have a cast of thousands and many, many scenes; others have only one or two players and a simple set. You just don't know until the movie starts, but it is always fascinating. Letting your movie play out allows for a deep stillness to be created inside of you. It's like letting a little repair team go deep into the body to create this wonderful feeling of restoration and balance. If you have the urge to speak, instead of acting on it, try to examine that urge, and the words behind it. Look at your words and thoughts the way you would look at fish swimming by you in a lake. Look at them as they appear, acknowledge them, then let the current carry them away.

If you have the urge to get up, try to examine your anxiousness, and the possible root of that, instead of acting on it. If you have the urge to scream, promise yourself you will give yourself that scream as soon as you are done, but right now, you want to understand what that scream is all about. The goal is to witness, but not to act. If you can witness without participating, engaging, reacting, identifying, or any other "ing," you have reached a very powerful place.

I have discovered that in my silence my intuitive process is much stronger and more connected. I can see a bigger picture and understand my reactions to the world around me. Without the clutter of my words, without the defensiveness of my words, without the seduction of my words, and without the armor of my words, a much healthier and more powerful me pokes its head out and takes over. It's amazing. Control has always been a big issue for me, and words have been a huge part of that mechanism. When I give that up, something so very wonderful happens. I can't predict what you will experience in your silence; I can only encourage you to give yourself a chance to have that experience. If you're feeling resistant to the idea, recognize that resistance is one of the clearest signs that very important lessons are waiting for you in that space.

THE "OTHER" CLEANSING RITUAL

In Europe, say the word "enema" and no one flinches. In the United States, say the word "enema" and everyone heads for the hills. This amazes me, especially since these same terrified people will chew countless chocolates, and guzzle all kinds of scary laxatives to encourage a bowel movement. But, let's face it, we all get embarrassed by this one. Many of us find the notion impossible.

People tell me, "I'll do anything on this fast, but I won't do an enema." I tell them, "Fine." And that's what I need to tell you right now. No one is going to force you to have an enema. That choice is yours and yours alone. However, I also need to let you know something else: everybody who overcomes their aversion to enemas and uses them during the fast calls me to thank me for encouraging them. Why? Because it makes you feel 100 percent better. Let me explain why.

As you now know, when you go on a juice fast, you are not putting any solid food into your stomach. Since your body doesn't have any new fiber to kick out of the system, it can turn its focus to the express transportation and evacuation of toxins. Round 'em up, and get 'em out. But the absence of solid food in the stomach also shuts off the complex mechanisms that produce bowel movements. It doesn't happen to everybody, but most people who are fasting will not have a bowel movement by Day 2 or Day 3. Here's the problem: there is still a lot of waste lingering in the colon. If the waste just sits there during the fast, your body could reabsorb some of the toxins that were heading for the exit. It also makes you feel weighty and logy—constipated. If you use an enema, the toxins are evacuated quickly and the system is cleared in a most healthy way.

Enema may be a scary word, but the process is really very gentle. Let me tell you how it's done, then you can make the decision as you see fit.

Enema bags can be purchased in most drugstores. They're usually sold as combination enema/douche bags. The first thing you do is fill the bag with lightly warmed water (test it on your wrist for comfort, the way you would test a baby's bottle) and the juice of half a lemon per quart of water you use.

Hang the filled bag on a nozzle in your bathtub. Remove your clothing and lie down in the empty tub. Let yourself relax. Once you have gotten comfortable, insert the end of the hose into your anus, using a little vitamin E oil to make the insertion easy. Do not use Vaseline. Now, slowly let the contents of the bag come into your body and fill you up a little bit. If you feel a little pressure in the beginning, try to breathe through it with short, firm exhalations.

Try to hold on to everything in your system for five to ten minutes if you can. Eight minutes would be perfect. Now get up, sit on the toilet, relax your sphincter muscles, and let the toxins leave your system. You did it!

I have read that human beings store five to ten pounds of waste in the colon that never gets out. It just keeps getting reabsorbed. You're not going to get that out with a simple enema, but you are going to start the process. Some day, you might consider going to a colonic therapist for a deeper cleaning. In the meantime, enjoy the energy pickup and other health benefits of this time-honored cleansing process. To the Europeans, using enemas on a fairly regular basis is a simple matter of health. We could all learn a lot from their attitude.

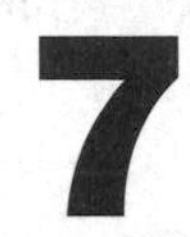

Exercises for a Spiritual Journey

The healing exercises included in this program will bring a wide range of benefits to your body, mind, and spirit without tiring you out. I think you will find that some of these exercises are absolutely invigorating, enabling you to find quick energy and strength. Some will help calm you down—particularly when you're feeling stress; some will help you balance the body and the spirit; and some will help you move through difficult emotional passages. All of these exercises are gentle and safe, and all of them make a tremendous difference during the fast.

Many of the people I've worked with have made some of these exercises a regular part of their day-to-day life, even when they are not fasting. This is particularly true for people who have never exercised regularly in the past, but it is also surprisingly common among exercise fanatics who scoffed at my gentler exercises when I first suggested them.

During your fast days, resist the urge to do any exercises except the ones included in this book. As you read through this material, all I ask is that, regardless of your knowledge and experience with exercise and fitness, try to stay open to bringing something new into your life.

EXERCISE #1: BREATH WORK

When I talk about breath work, I don't mean brushing, flossing, and gargling with Scope. I'm talking about amazing exercises that will help you tune in, focus on, and develop your greatest gift—breathing. Tension, apprehension, anger, serenity, and happiness all have a startling effect on breathing patterns. Did you ever become so tense that you noticed that you were holding your breath? When we are nervous or upset, without realizing it, we stop breathing in a natural way. These distressed breathing patterns can become hardened habits and part of who we are.

Breathing exercises are an honored ancient method of balancing the emotional, spiritual, and physical sides of our nature. Learning how to breathe—how to fully, consciously breathe—will support your fast and energize the process of becoming new. This is why we will take time to do special breath work at various times during the three days of fasting.

Every time we inhale, our breath sends oxygen—the message of life—to every cell in the body. Every time we exhale, our breath takes out the trash—carbon monoxide—creating ideal conditions for growth and life. Breathing is also our best natural defense against germs, disease, and bacteria. We too easily take this constant vital cleansing process for granted and often ignore it completely. Conscious breathing is an essential ingredient in a detox program.

No one would ever try to go a day without breathing, yet so many people *do* go for days, months, and even years without breathing *well*—without using the gift of breath to fully deliver all of its fuel to the body. What about you? How deeply do you breathe? How slowly do you breathe? How fully do you breathe? And have you ever even *noticed*? Have you noticed, for example, that when you are feeling anxiety or fear, and your mind is racing with thought, your breaths become short, high in your chest, and barely "in your body"? Have you noticed that on other days, when you're feeling more calm, connected, grounded, and at peace, your breath is so much deeper, full of tone and substance? Do you sometimes get so upset that you literally forget to breathe? Does your breath come out in little pathetic sighs? Do you shortchange your breathing? When you breathe, do you have a harder time breathing in (accepting) or breathing out (letting go)?

Often the only thing between you and a specific action or non-action is your breath. You breathe, for example, while you decide what to say or not say. Sometimes the only thing you have left between you and your fear is your breath. In short, the only thing between you and the rest of the world is your breath. You need to be aware of it, learn how to use it, and learn how to protect it.

Learning how to breathe has changed my life, and I know it will change yours. It has brought me into consciousness and into complete aliveness. It has rejuvenated my entire body, organ by organ. As a special bonus, it has served as my "in-house cosmetic surgeon," making my face look ten years younger without costing a dime! The more life I give to my breath, the more life it gives back to me.

No matter what is happening to me, I know I have my breath and that it will support me. I use breathing exercises to push through anxieties, uncertainty, sadness, and loss; I also use them to accentuate and celebrate the positives in life. My breath is what grounds me and it is what *is* me. When I am not paying attention to my breath, I am not paying attention to my life.

We literally live our lives one breath at a time. What could be more beautiful, more poetic, more simple, and more perfect. During these three days of detoxification I want you to indulge yourself with your breath. Indulgence begins with awareness, which is where we have just begun. The rest is easy, and the breathing exercises you will discover throughout the three-day program will show you how.

EXERCISE #2: WALKING MAGIC

At least once a day during your fast, I want you to take a long walk, and I want you to find something uplifting and magical in that walk. Walking is a chance to get more fully energized, to speed up elimination, and to accelerate the cleansing process by encouraging the release of toxins. Last, but far from least, a walk gives you a chance to get out of your head and into the world, to take note of all of the life that surrounds you and how you are connected to that life.

One of the primary goals of fasting is to find the life inside us, but there is also so much life *outside*, just waiting to be experienced.

I always carry a little pouch with me when I go for my walks. I use this pouch to collect things I might find along the way—rocks, leaves, twigs, shells, flowers. These trinkets keep me connected to nature, and help continue my walk long after the physical act has ended. When my walk is done, I often place these objects on my altar or save them in my journal, and I encourage you to do the same thing.

How quickly will you walk? That's up to you. Some days you will be brisk, other days you will be slow; some days you will glide, other days you will skip. You don't want to run, and you probably won't feel like running anyway. If you're a hard-core athlete who is always pushing her/his body, please fight the urge. I don't believe in pumping and pushing all the time. I believe that the body, in its infinite wisdom, knows what it needs each day, and that those needs are always slightly different. I tell people, let your legs lead the way, not your head. Drink with your eyes, but give your mind a chance to rest.

To help your mind rest, keep yourself present, and keep your insides connected to the wonders outside of you, I have a special walking meditation. I'd like you to use this meditation each day you take your special walk (see below).

The Walking Meditation

The traditions of Asian religions have always understood the significance of "Walking Meditation." Use this meditation to help you connect more fully with your world:

As you take each step of your walk, let the weight of your body press firmly into the ground. Look at everything you pass, and, if only for a moment, try to become each of the things you see. Think to yourself: I am the bushes; I am the rocks, the pebbles, the concrete; I am the grass. Become the flower you see, the dog you see, the little child you see. Give special time to the things that capture your imagination or your heart the most. Stare at these things (unless, of course, they are people), study them, then become them. For just a moment, can you experience what they are experiencing? As you continue your walk, let yourself open more and more to the world that is passing by you. Let the world make strong impressions on your memory. Let yourself experience this world as more than a blur. Use all of your senses. Make everything you see feel welcome inside of you. Your fasting time will be a time of opening, a time of many new beginnings. Your walks are a way to practice your welcome. To let go of fear and invite in all possibility and a new sense of life and vitality. Tell your spirit it is completely free to wander, to play, and to seek the infinite.

EXERCISE #3: YOGA

The word *yoga* implies union: the union of a clear, peaceful mind and a sound, healthy body. Yoga balances the mind, the body, and the spirit through the use of stretching, breathing technique, and special postures. During a yoga session, you can sweat, tone, stretch, and relax. When we get tense and tight, a twisted spine is a twisted mind; yoga will straighten you out. Through yoga, we reopen and remember ourselves.

Yoga makes the spine more supple and available. It cleanses, clears, strengthens, revitalizes, rejuvenates, and harmonizes all the negative patterning in the system. It illuminates beauty, it changes dietary habits, it restores healthy elimination, and it even transforms facial expressions (wrinkles go away!). It's a powerful practice, but it's also so very gentle. For me, yoga does it all. (See the ten yoga postures in Appendix A, pages 223–35, for a simple and enlivening routine.)

EXERCISE #4: SCREAMING OUT THE OLD, SCREAMING IN THE NEW

During your fast, I want you to practice releasing your old voice and your old ways. There are three brand-new things I want you to be able to do with your voice.

1. Learn to speak so that your expression is clear and your intention is heard.
2. Start saying things you've never said before.
3. Stop saying the same old things in the same old ways.

Screaming is the Roto-Rooter of the voice. It rids the voice of excuses, and it puts an end to procrastination. Most important of all, by connecting us to two simple words—"yes" and "no"—it connects us to our greatest power. Cleaning out and staying clean means learning to say no to all of the toxic things you have allowed into your body, your mind, and your life. It means saying no to bad food, bad habits, bad jobs, bad relationships, bad etc., etc., etc. If you have said yes all your life when you wanted to say no, you have filled up with things that make you fed up. You are probably aching to change that, but "no" is such a hard word to say. That's why we have to practice, and practice really loud.

During the fast, I encourage you to do a screaming exercise that builds and strengthens the "no" muscle. This may sound extreme, but sometimes we need to go to the extreme before we can find a comfortable middle ground. If you've had a hard time saying no all your life, you're going to need that scream to break through your barriers and inhibitions. You're probably feeling pretty victimized, and the only way to overcome that is with strength.

Part of the process of becoming new means finding, building, and using new parts of yourself. Appropriate screaming (into a pillow, on a deserted beach, in the woods, etc.) helps you feel your own strength. It tells the world you're not going to take it anymore, and it sends the same message to the deep insides of your self.

Then, watch out! Once you start saying no, there may be no stopping you. Everything that has made you feel powerless starts coming to the surface to get kicked out of your life. Suddenly, you're a warrior. You're not embarrassed anymore, you're not wishy-washy anymore, and you're not a victim anymore.

A second screaming exercise we'll be doing is the "yes" exercise. Once you've started to kick out the old, you're ready to welcome the new. You're ready to say yes to health, to vitality, to love, and to change. And this time, you get to choose. In the beginning, you need to scream your invitation really loud, to make sure that *you* really hear it, and feel it, and believe. Because you deserve it!

The first time I felt the power of "no!" it really felt like a miracle. I was sitting on the beach, thinking about my toxic office, and how it was slowly killing me. All of a sudden, this huge, spontaneous "No!" roared out of my mouth from deep within my body. I was totally embarrassed, and immediately looked around to see if anyone had been watching me. Fortunately, the beach was empty. So I screamed again. And again. And again. And again . . . When I woke up the next morning, I had no voice left. But I had gained something else: clarity. Within weeks, I left my job and left that toxic world behind.

The lesson I learned was simple and powerful: If you want to leave your toxic world behind, sometimes you need to shout it out, and if you want to bring a new, healthier world in, sometimes you need to shout it in with a strong positive "Yes!"

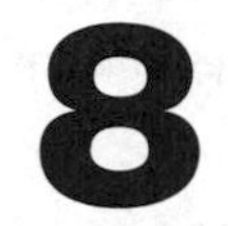

Setting the Stage

You don't have to star on Broadway to know that the hardest work has been done long before the curtain rises on opening night. Well, it's the same thing with the 3-Day Energy Fast. You need to do a run-through in your head and prepare spiritually and emotionally. You need to prepare your body. You should also prepare your family, and maybe your friends and coworkers too. And you are going to have a fair amount of practical preparation—the nuts and bolts of this three-day adventure. That means making lists and planning your shopping for fruits and vegetables. You will need to shop for your skin brush, your bath salts, and various comfort items. If you don't already have them, you'll have to buy, or borrow, a juicer and a blender. I'll discuss each of these in detail shortly. You've got a lot to do before you are ready to start.

Ideally, the only thing you want to have to focus on during your three days of fasting is: your three days of fasting. Yet I realize that for most of us, if not *all* of us, this is simply not possible. Even those of us who don't have children, pets, or high-pressure careers still lead very complicated lives. That is just the way the world has become, and it is one of the reasons that taking this three-day healing opportunity is so important. Even if you can't isolate yourself for three days, the more you can simplify your life during the fast, the more you will free yourself to stay focused on this extraordinary opportunity, and to maximize its benefits. The key to simplification is planning and preparation.

BEFORE YOU START, READ EVERYTHING IN THIS BOOK

The program in this book actually has three distinct phases:

- a prefast (two to three days before the fast)
- the 3-Day Fast
- a break-fast (one to two days after the fast)

Before you begin the prefast, carefully read through all three phases of this program. Right now, you need to familiarize yourself with the program. Reading everything carefully will prepare you for what you will be doing, feeling, eating, and drinking.

This program is very straightforward and is really easy to follow if you take the time to understand the simple things that need to be done *before* you plunge forward. Walk through it in your mind and get comfortable with everything that is new or unusual to you. Take notes and reread anything that seems the least bit confusing, complicated, or unclear. Think about special things you can do to make and keep everything simple for yourself.

GOING SHOPPING

Once you have familiarized yourself with the complete program, you need to establish everything that you will be needing, and you need to start planning your shopping trips.

To make this program as easy for you as possible, do as much of your shopping as possible *before you begin your prefast*. Aside from the program items, this also includes anything you, your family, or your pets might need for the next week. Now is the time to stock the pantry, the fridge, and the closets. You do not want to find yourself wandering the aisles of your favorite supermarket once this program begins. You do not want to have to run to the drugstore, and you don't want to be at the mall. You don't need the temptation. You don't need the confusion. You don't need to be losing precious energy. And you don't need to be spending your sacred time involved in these activities.

KITCHEN ITEMS

The kitchen is where you have the most work to do. So let's start there and list some of the most basic items you're going to need. I call this the Master Accessory List:

1. a vegetable juicer to make all of your fresh juices
2. a blender to make your special daily Morning Drink
3. a good knife, strong and sharp, to cut all of your fruits and vegetables for juicing
4. several large bowls for your fruits and vegetables
5. clear plastic wrap to cover bowls
6. one large pot to prepare your broth
7. plastic refrigerator bags (1-quart size, Ziploc or similar) to store prepped fruits and vegetables
8. a cutting board
9. airtight bottles (three or four, preferably glass) to store left-over juice

Perhaps you already have these items at home. If you don't, now is the time to buy them. You could, of course, also borrow many of these items from friends, family, or neighbors. If you think your fast will be more than just a one-time event, or if you are hoping to incorporate elements of the fast into your life on a regular basis, this could be the right time to make some basic purchases.

PRODUCE

Right now, you may feel as though you would like to go shopping every morning of the fast for the freshest produce, but this may not be how you are going to feel once you start fasting. Before you start the prefast, make a comprehensive list of the food you're going to need. You know how fresh the fruits and veggies are in your supermarket or organic produce department, and you'll have a sense of how long various items will keep. You may be able to do all your shopping at once. At the very least, you can do most of your shopping ahead of time.

As you read through the juice menus in this book, one of the first things you will notice is that some of the juice drinks vary according to your personal desires, and the seasonal availability of produce. This means that you need to make some choices, and you need to make these choices *before* the fast begins. I wish this could be a more spontaneous process, but once the fast begins, you will be very happy knowing that all of your decisions have already been made, and all of your ingredients have already been assembled. So look at all of the juice recipes, make your choices, and write down all of the ingredients you will need for each day on your Master Food List. Don't rely on memory when you shop, and don't try to wing it.

Here are a few helpful hints. If you can afford to splurge a little right now, buy some extra produce. This way, you can cover the possibility of any mistakes, spills, or other surprises (like Fido drinking your breakfast). It's also a good idea to pad your food list with surplus ingredients for your vegetable broth and your other juices. Better to have leftovers than not to have enough. Don't forget to get plenty of herbal tea (loose, or in bags), lots of lemons, and lots and lots of spring water.

Break your Master Food List up into three sections, titled as follows:

- For the Prefast I Will Need . . .
- For the Fast I Will Need . . .
- For the Break-Fast I Will Need . . .

THE SPECIAL INGREDIENTS

- acidophilus (a friendly bacteria culture used here in its dairy-free powder form)
- flaxseed oil (be sure it's fresh)
- tamari sauce (organic and wheat-free)

You should be able to find these special ingredients at most health-food stores and even supermarkets, so please don't omit any of them unless you really have to.

ALWAYS CREATE A SETTING

Typically, we eat a lot of food every day, but very few of us pay close attention to the process. We wolf down breakfast over the kitchen sink, we gobble french fries as we maneuver through crosstown traffic, and we inhale dinner half-mesmerized by the evening news. It has to be very different during your days of fasting, and it begins by creating a special setting. During the fast, every glass of juice, every bowl of broth, and every cup of tea is an event to be celebrated. They are all special and they are all doing something special to your body. Creating a unique setting gives all of your meals this feeling.

Start by finding yourself a really great glass. Maybe it will be a beautiful piece of crystal, maybe it will be a family heirloom, or maybe it will just be the favorite glass you already have. You are also going to need a special bowl and spoon for your broth (plastic spoons are a no-no), and a great mug for your warm drinks. Get a lovely place mat, and find a small vase for fresh flowers if this appeals to you. You will definitely need a comfortable chair. *Never* eat standing up.

OTHER ACCESSORIES

The accessories in the following list will enhance the program for you. Make sure you don't leave them out.

- **Art supplies**
  You should have paper, pencils, and crayons or markers. You might also want other art supplies to play with during your fasting days.

- **Bath items**
  Get a good natural fiber skin brush that is not too abrasive. You might also want a loofah mitt. You're also going to need

Epsom salts or the fragrant bath salts of your choice. The rule of thumb is at least one large handful of salts per bath, but I like to use two or three handfuls. Don't forget your special essences for the bath (bath oils, or essential oils and fragrance-free emulsifiers to make your own bath oils), your "mood items" (candles, etc.), and any bath toys that might be fun.

- **Music**
  Be sure you have gentle music that you find soothing and uplifting as well as a stereo, boom box, or personal Walkman to play them on.

- **Food for thought**
  You are going on a spiritual journey. This is a wonderful time to read some of the extraordinary spiritual literature that has inspired so many people to change their lives and strengthen their commitments.

- **Comfortable clothes**
  Be sure to have loose-fitting, comfortable clothing to exercise in and to wear around the house during the fast. You don't want to be confined by tight jeans or expensive designer garb. This is a time to feel relaxed.

- **Special cleansing items**
  I encourage you to get an inexpensive enema/douche bag if you don't already have one.

- **Your journal**
  You want to get a notebook or journal that feels really special to you.

- **Loving things for your sacred space and altar**
  Have you already filled your sacred space and altar? If there is anything you want to add, now is the time to do so.

- **Miscellaneous items**
  Do you want a special pen for your journal? A beautiful spoon for your broth? A waterproof radio for your bath? This is a time to be generous and loving to yourself, even to spoil yourself a little.

LOVING AND PREPARING YOUR FOOD

Once you have completed all your shopping, the time has come to create a relationship with the wonderful and colorful fruits and veggies that will be nourishing you during your fasting journey. Before you start washing, peeling, or putting anything in the refrigerator, the very first thing you should do is gather all of your produce together in a large, beautiful pile on your kitchen table or kitchen counter. Make believe you're shooting a family photo and arrange all of your produce lovingly to show off its bounty. Now stop, take a few deep breaths, and look at everything before you.

Are you still concerned about making it through your three-day fast? Are you worried you'll be hungry? Are you afraid your body won't be getting enough nourishment? Then take a long look at how much extraordinary, healthful sustenance you will be giving to your body during your fast. Just look at it. Stare at it. Let yourself get lost in it. The sight of this enormous collection should be overwhelming. Take a picture of it with your mind's eye and commit the image to memory. You might even want to take a real photograph to have on your altar for support. Remember this program is not about starvation, but about creating new life. I hope that you can start believing that now.

Until you begin prepping, fill your large bowls with your fresh fruits and vegetables and decorate your kitchen with these bowls so you feel constantly surrounded by all of your beautiful produce. Refrigerate any fragile produce, but also use your bowls (and plastic wrap to cover those bowls, if necessary) in the refrigerator. Brown bags full of produce are not very exciting or appetizing. On the other hand, beautiful bowls brimming with gorgeous produce can be absolutely inspiring.

A Short Prayer

Before I do any physical prep work, I usually like to say a little prayer over the fruit and vegetables. I ask them to cleanse me, to be friendly to my body, and to minimize my discomfort through the detox. Sometimes my prayer turns into a little chat with my food, and it always seems to help. Talking to your produce may, at first, strike you as a little bit fruity. But if you can get past the awkwardness, you will start to develop an important and very different kind of relationship with these foods. By spending time with your fruits and vegetables, you are inviting them to come into your system and work with you to bring health and life. The process begins with the fast, but it can continue throughout the course of your life.

THE PHYSICAL PREP

Buy it, squeeze it, pour it, and drink it up. It would be nice if you could prep all your produce for juicing at one time. But you can't because it might spoil. However, since you've done all your shopping, before you start each of your three days of actual fasting, you will find it more efficient to have all of your fruits and vegetables *for that one day* thoroughly washed, counted out, peeled, or pitted when necessary and ready to throw into your juicer, blender, or soup pot. The best time to do this is either first thing in the morning, or the night before.

The last night of the prefast is a particularly important evening for preparation. As you approach the fast, you will be partially excited, anticipating what is to come, and partially dreading it. You might be fearing failure, and concerned about wanting food. Or you might be fearing the symptoms of your cleaning, worrying "Will I feel yucky?" At a time like this, it really helps to be close to all the foods you have assembled for the fast.

The easiest way to stay organized is to read over the menus at the beginning of each fast day, and the recipes at the back of the book. Then make your juice choices, and assemble your ingredients for the day *one recipe at a time*. When you have gathered together all of the fruits and/or vegetables a recipe calls for, and everything has been sliced, diced, and fully prepped for juicing, blending or boiling, place these ingredients in one of your quart-sized plastic bags and label the bag clearly. For example, your first bag would say: Morning Drink, Day 1. The next bag you prepare would say: Mid-Morning Drink, Day 1, etc., etc. When you have done all of your food preparation, you should have a separate bag for *every meal* of the day. The one exception will be made in preparing the ingredients for your broth. I recommend you make all of your broth at one time, so all of the ingredients for five days of broth should be assembled in one larger bag (or several quart-sized bags).

Do not put special ingredients, such as the acidophilus, tamari, or flaxseed oil into any of your plastic bags—these ingredients are to go directly into your blender, your glass, or your soup pot during your final preparation.

I know this sounds like a lot of bags and a lot of work, but you'll discover that it's actually easier than cooking dinner. Doing a day's worth of preparation at a time really makes a huge difference once the fast begins. I don't want you giving up on your fast because you were too tired to peel, slice, and dice. But I've seen it happen, and I know that this is the best way to insure that it doesn't happen to *you*. During the prefast, you will have a lot of energy just thinking about the wonderful changes that are soon to come into your life. The best thing you can do right now is to use that energy to get ready.

ESTABLISH A RELATIONSHIP WITH YOUR JUICER

Don't wait till Day 1 of the fast to start making juice. If you've never before used an electric vegetable juicer, now is the time to learn some of the basics of juicing. The absolute best way to do that is by making yourself, your family, and your friends some fantastic fresh juice. Since every juicer is different, you need to learn some specifics about the machine you now have. How do you get it ready? How do you clean it when you're done? How often do you need to clean it? What kinds of noises does it make? What is the optimal size for the pieces of fruit and vegetables you put in your machine? Are there any fruits or vegetables it can't handle? Read your manufacturer's instruction booklet carefully and practice, practice, practice.

MAKING NECESSARY ARRANGEMENTS

Even if you don't have to go to work during your three days of fasting, you will still have daily concerns that require your attention. Newspapers, mail, and packages may need to be picked up;

bills need to be paid; plants may need to be watered; dogs may need to be walked; children may need to be carpooled. During your three days of fasting, you can't turn the demands of the outside world off completely, but there are certainly many things you can do to keep it at arm's length.

Now is the time to think about the many demands of your day-to-day life and anticipate how they will affect your schedule during your three days of fasting. Make a comprehensive list of what needs to be done and problems that could arise. How can your many demands be simplified? Your goal is to minimize disruptions and interruptions during your three days of fasting.

PREPARING YOUR FAMILY

If you have a partner, children, or even a roommate, get their cooperation. You want to arm them with as much information as possible from the very beginning so there are no conflicts later on. The best way to do this is to sit down with these people *before you begin your prefast* and explain clearly what it is you are going to be doing. Give them an opportunity to ask questions so they don't feel excluded from your life.

Here's one very big rule for you, your friends, and your family to understand and respect: *The less you are around everyone else's food while you are fasting, the better.*

You also want to stay far away from the kitchen table during their mealtimes, and that means telling everyone way in advance that they shouldn't expect you to join them or ask you to join them. Even the smell of food can make you uncomfortable, and it is something you just don't need to experience if you can avoid it. Their mealtimes are a great time for you to take a bath, rest in your bedroom, or go for a walk. You can rejoin everybody after they have eaten and the table has been cleared.

PREPARING YOUR COWORKERS

If you have to go back to work on Day 2 or Day 3 of your fast, prepare your office mates ahead of time. You don't really want to keep your fast a secret unless you absolutely have to. You may want some extra time to be alone, and if you can let your coworkers know what you are doing, they might be very helpful and supportive. They might think twice before they eat bagels and candy bars and grilled Reuben sandwiches right in front of your face. They are more likely to respect you for being able to fast.

Keeping secrets is another way we make ourselves toxic. Keeping secrets creates stress, stress creates acids, acids create havoc, etc., etc. So tell your office mates if you can, and be proud of your decision to fast.

PREPARING TO SLOW DOWN

If you have to choose one mantra for these three days, it should be the word *slow*. So much in life happens way too quickly. We eat too fast, we drive too fast, we talk too fast, and we make love too fast. Moments after we wake up each morning it seems like we're out the door; we rush through the day to get everything done, then we race home to grab some dinner and catch an hour of television. We try to process information at the speed of light, and we say "yes" and "no" before we ever think about the consequences. Fasting is the antidote to all of this. To fast is to slow our life down. The process brings us into our body, it brings us into our feelings, and it connects us to the universe. We become more aware of our posture, our breathing, our muscles and skin tone, our voice, our senses, our thoughts and conflicts, our pain, and our pleasure.

Slowing down brings you to your center, and it brings you into a sense of aliveness that is genuinely spiritual.

Right now, you may feel as though you want to get your three-day fast over with as quickly as possible. That is not how fasting works. You do not want to rush these days. You don't want to be staring at your watch and ticking off the minutes and hours. I actually take my watch off whenever I fast. Every aspect of this program has been designed to be done slowly—the exercises, the rituals, the meditations, even the meals. You want to rest, reflect, pamper yourself, nourish yourself, and heal. You want to be completely in the moment, drinking your glorious juices one sip at a time. You want to be savoring the pleasures of your baths, immersing yourself in your rituals and relishing the specialness of these three days. And the most important clock during these three days is your internal clock—the only clock that really knows when your body needs rest, when it needs nourishment, when it needs exercise, and when it needs sleep.

PREPARING TO LET GO

Going on a three-day fast means putting your normal life on hold for a while, particularly if this is your first ritual fast. You're not going to be following your regular routines, and you're not going to have your normal diet. You're going to be taking a vacation from the life you have always lived—the life you have become very comfortable living (even if it is not a comfortable way of life). And right now, you don't know how you're going to feel when you get back from this vacation. You might want to go back to the life you have been living *exactly* as you have been living it. You might want to go back to the same life, but with a new understanding. Or you might want to make *all kinds of changes* in your life—changes you may have never even dreamed of. The most important thing right now is to stay open to *any* and every possibility.

Preparing for the 3-Day Detox is, more than anything, preparing to let go, so that everything your mind, body, and spirit needs for healing can unfold naturally.

The first thing you're going to be letting go of is food. For some people that may be the hardest thing; for others it may be the easiest. Now is the time to start to really look at food and what it means to you. What will it feel like not to have your favorite foods for a few days—that first cup of morning coffee, your morning bagel, the diet sodas, the spoonful of Häagen-Dazs that soothes you before bedtime. You need to think about your favorite foods—even the ones you thought were healthy—and prepare yourself to say good-bye. Not good-bye forever, but good-bye for now. I'm not asking you to pass judgment on them right now. That isn't necessary. By the time your fast is complete, you will have learned naturally what foods are good for you and what foods are not so good for you, and you will make decisions then about what you want to do with all this new information. The important thing right now is to fully acknowledge the role these foods have in your life today, and prepare for your good-byes.

During your fasting days, you are also going to be letting go of the many people in your life. You're not actually going to be saying good-bye to anybody—you're not even going away. Your family will still be there. Your friends will still be your friends. But from the time you begin your preparation till the time your fast is over, your relationships with these people are going to be very different. Your days of fasting are days devoted to your own personal healing and transformation, and the people in your life won't be able to reach you in the same way and they will not be able to count on you in the same way. And you will not be wanting the same things from them for these three days. Even if these changes are only very temporary, they are significant changes. You need to be prepared, and these people need to be prepared too. And there's more. You're going to be letting go of schedules, routines, old habits, expectations, and preconceived notions. It's a lot to let go of, and you need to start now.

The Prefast

To help your body adjust to the changes in your diet and ease you into this program gently, it is *essential* that you follow a prefast for at least two or three days before your three-day fast begins. I realize that right now, the desire to "cut to the chase" may be nagging at you, or even hounding you, and I want to reassure you that you will be starting your fast soon, very soon. But if you are going to fast, you need to do it right, and that means doing a prefast. A proper prefast will ease your body through the transition from solid foods to juice, and it will do this with a minimum amount of discomfort and shock to the system. A prefast will also ease your mind and contribute to your emotional and spiritual state of readiness by getting you focused on the many changes that are soon to come.

The prefast diet suggestions in this program are fairly simple, and you need to follow them as closely as possible for *forty-eight hours* before you begin your fast. If you are fasting for the first time, if you are very nervous about the fasting process, or if you have unhealthy or extreme eating habits, then I recommend prefasting for seventy-two hours.

If you are really hooked on sugar, caffeine, alcohol, wheat, or any other substance, it may be too difficult for you to eliminate these abruptly, and you may need to give yourself extra time—perhaps even a week or more—to disconnect from these foods in a sane and manageable way. Anyone wishing to follow this program *must* prefast for a minimum of twenty-four hours. If, for whatever reason, you cannot meet this minimum requirement, do not proceed with the program at this time. Instead, wait until a better window of opportunity arises in your schedule.

PREFAST NO-NOS

Let's start by talking once again about what you *shouldn't* eat. During, and for at least twenty-four hours prior to, the start of your fast, stay away from:

sugar

caffeine (tea, coffee, cola)

oils

wheat

alcohol

meat

dairy products (cheese, milk, butter, or anything that is made with these ingredients)

Now that's a lot to abstain from. We're talking no candy, gum, sugar-sweetened baked goods, or sugar-sweetened beverages. No coffee, caffeinated teas, or colas. No bread, cake, or pie that's made with wheat. No beer, wine, hard liquor, or alcohol-flavored anything. No beef, pork, chicken, or fish. No milk, cream, butter, cheese, or yogurt. These short lists aren't comprehensive, but if you read your labels carefully, you will figure out where the seven culprits may be hiding. You will also learn something very important about some of the secret ingredients that lurk in the shadows of your daily diet.

Asking you to eliminate sugar, caffeine, wheat, alcohol, oil, meat, and dairy products from your diet is asking a lot—even if it's only for a very short time. You're probably not going to be able to do this perfectly. You need to try as hard as you can to be as "good" as you can. To make it easier, you can do it in stages. Start by eliminating meat four or five days before the fast. The next day, take out dairy products and oils. Then take out wheat and sugar. Remember: You are doing this for you, not for me. And it will make the fasting process much easier on your system.

WHAT *CAN* YOU EAT?

Overall, I recommend that you limit your diet to vegetables, soups (dairy-free), salads, and fruits. With a little ingenuity and imagination you should be able to make these choices go a long way with respect to variety and taste.

Try to eat your fruits and vegetables at different times. Ideally, it would be great if you could wait at least two hours before switching from one to the other. Despite what we have all learned from our parents and teachers, most fruits and vegetables do not mix well digestively. This conflict slows digestion down and slows you down, and you are going to start feeling particularly sensitive to this on a limited prefast diet.

Here are some more specific suggestions:

Breakfast

For breakfast every morning of your prefast, you can have any fresh fruits you like, with the exception of oranges and bananas—both are too acidic. Not much room to get creative? You'd be surprised at what you can do with some of the exotic fruits that you can now find on supermarket shelves. And you may also be pleasantly surprised at how light and energetic your body feels when you start your day with food it doesn't have to labor intensively to digest. Your mind may be saying "No, no, no," but your body is already going to start saying "Yes, yes, yes," and you are going to like the way that feels. To drink, have herbal tea, or better yet, warm water with lemon. If you prefer, miso soup is an acceptable breakfast alternative, but it is either fruits *or* miso, not both.

Lunch

For lunch every afternoon of your prefast, make yourself a wonderful salad of freshly mixed raw vegetables. Or you can have a combination of raw and steamed vegetables. Try to make it colorful and creative, and if you can, organic. Always clean your produce well before you eat it, and feel free to have as much vegetable salad as you like. Some good choices: broccoli, yellow squash, zucchini, butternut or acorn squash, green beans, snow peas, asparagus. I call it a rainbow plate.

If you have a favorite oil-free salad dressing that isn't loaded with preservatives or other scary ingredients, use it, but I would suggest moderation. Once again, keep your fruits and vegetables separate. For that reason, it's a good idea to wait at least two hours between breakfast and lunch. And try not to nibble in between.

Dinner

In the summer months, you may feel like another raw vegetable salad for dinner, but having a generous serving of steamed vegetables will definitely make your daily prefast menu a little more interesting. If you like, season your steamed vegetables with fat-free tamari. You can also use your oil-free dressing for your salad or your steamed veggies. Since your dinner may not be as exciting as what you are used to, be sure to use the freshest and best of everything that *is* available to you. It is okay to have potato or rice with your prefast lunches and/or dinners, but don't eat potatoes or rice on the last night of your prefast. On the last night, you need to keep yourself very clean, and these complex carbohydrates will get in the way.

The "Mono" Diet

If it appeals to you, you may want to try a slightly different approach to prefasting, something known as a "mono" diet. A mono diet, quite simply, is a diet of only one type of food—such as *only* grapes, *only* melons, *only* apples, or *only* green salad—for all of your meals. You might want to try this for the last day of your prefast, or, if you're feeling really courageous, you might want to try this for several days. It's a great precleanser, and it will also help you build valuable food discipline. And yes, technically speaking, eating *only* chocolate is also a mono diet, but in this mono diet, your only options are fruits or vegetables.

If you are going to try a mono diet, remember not to mix fruits with vegetables. If, for example, you start with apples, stay with just apples. If you start with veggies, stick with just veggies—veggies for breakfast, veggies for lunch, veggies for dinner, and veggies for any snacking in between meals.

If you want to go on a mono diet, either grapes or watermelon are good choices. On the vegetable side, asparagus or yellow summer squash are terrific.

And this is very important: If you are hypoglycemic, or sensitive to sugar, I would advise that you don't go on a mono fruit diet. An entire day of just fruits will overwhelm your system, and it could make you sick. If you have a sugar sensitivity, but still really want to try a mono diet, go with green salads or steamed vegetables.

"WATER, WATER, EVERYWHERE"

And I'm talking about drinking plenty of it—a *minimum* of eight 8-ounce glasses of natural springwater every day of the prefast. Water is one of the best friends your body ever had. It's one of nature's great purifiers, and it's entirely fat- and calorie-free. During the prefast, drinking lots of water will help activate the cleansing process, a process that will be continued with fresh juices and broths once your fast begins.

You want to use water during your prefast to help keep flushing toxins from your system around the clock. But let me tell you about something I know from experience. In the interest of getting a sound night's sleep right now, you might consider drinking the majority of your water in the first half of the day, and gradually tapering off toward evening. You know your body best, and you know how much water you can drink at night, and how late you can drink it, before you have to start taking the shuttle to the bathroom every twenty minutes. So work with your body to maximize the possibilities of both cleansing and a sound sleep.

Remember, you do *not* want to drink carbonated water, not even naturally carbonated mineral water, during your prefast or your fast. Although these various sparkling waters are usually friendly to the body, they can really bother the stomach during the fasting and detox process.

STAY POSITIVE

Do everything you can to stay positive and excited about the change in your daily menu. This is a bold adventure, and you need to treat it that way. Instead of moaning and groaning about the things you miss, why not pretend that you have just washed up on a desert island and that you are truly grateful to Mother Nature for all of the simple, beautiful, natural delicacies she has supplied to keep you alive and well? This is a time to connect to the most simple and important things in your life, and that includes the natural foods that are in such abundance. Think about how happy you are going to be when you lose what I call "wheat bloat" and your stomach looks and feels flat. If none of this works, you can always remind yourself that you're only doing this for a few days, not forever.

GIVE YOUR THOUGHTS THE VALUE THEY DESERVE BY USING YOUR JOURNAL

Be sure to set aside time during your prefast for writing, thinking, and meditating on your thoughts. Give your thoughts the value and weight they deserve. Now is the time to begin to ask yourself some important questions—questions you may wish to ponder during the fast. Why are you choosing to fast? What are some of the goals you hope to achieve—what are your short-term fasting goals and what are your long-term life goals? What are some of the patterns in your life you hope to change or eliminate? If you already have answers to some of these questions, write your answers down in your journal. If these questions stir many feelings inside of you, write about these feelings in your journal.

This is your chance to look back over your life for the last three years. Look at the area of work, look at the area of food, look at the area of relationships, and look at the area of spiritual growth. See where you have come from and see where you wish to go. How can you use the fast to empower your new dreams and vision for yourself? Create a picture of that new person you wish to be and make a list in your journal of all the ways you want to change physically, emotionally, and spiritually.

Now is also the time to psyche yourself up for the transformation available to you through this spiritual juice-fasting. You are doing a beautiful and sacred thing for yourself. How does this make you feel? Be aware that you are about to begin a cleansing process that can lead the way to the restoration of your body's natural integrity, balance, and well-being. Your body and your spirit want to be healthy, and you are giving them a chance to cleanse, to heal. When you are consciously aligned with this process, cocreating it with your higher self, miracles can happen. Allow yourself to feel the excitement that comes with all of this possibility, and write about your feelings in your journal.

Be certain to enter the current date with all of your journal entries so you can use the journal to remember how you are, and how you change, day by day.

THE "GOOD-BYE" RITUAL

On the last day of your prefast there is a little ritual I would like you to perform to help send you on your journey. It begins by sitting down, getting quiet, and thinking about all of the things you would like to change or let go of during your fast. Think about all of the behavior patterns that haven't served you well—eating patterns, relationship patterns, work habits, negative feelings, etc. Think about the things you do that you would like to do differently. Give yourself some time to create this list. Really reflect on this and allow yourself plenty of space to really travel through your interior, searching for emotional, physical, and spiritual issues you really want to let go of. What do you wish to be free of? How would you like to be different in the future? What would you like to say good-bye to? Try to be very specific. Your list might include items such as these:

"I fail to ask friends for what I need."

"I prioritize romance in an unhealthy way, losing sight of

other important relationships in my life for months at a time."

"I drink too much coffee."

"I eat my lunch too quickly at work, and I often eat at my desk instead of taking a break like I should."

"I always see the glass as half empty."

"I tend to overkill most of my job tasks, going way beyond what is expected of me."

"I don't let myself rest on the weekends unless I am totally exhausted or sick."

"I put too much salt on my food."

"I drive too fast on the highways."

"I am still trying to get approval from my family for who I am and what I do for a living."

"I never exercise."

"I spend too much money on clothes I never wear."

"I worry constantly about whether or not I have done my job well enough."

"I waste too much time on the telephone talking to people I really don't want to be talking to."

"I am very quick to judge and evaluate others."

One by one, write each of these things down on its own individual strip of paper. It is important to fully name each item, and the writing helps you do that. When you have finished, put all of these strips of paper in a little ceramic bowl.

Now, humbly offer these things up, one by one, by creating a small fire in your bowl. As the smoke rises, imagine all of these unhealthy patterns disappearing from your life in a puff of smoke. Now imagine that their leaving has created room in the deepest part of your body and your psyche for all of the growth, clarity, happiness, and dreams that you are intending to create on, and after, your three-day fast. In your exalted state, you can even bless those old habits and patterns on their journey out of your life, knowing that they were in your life for a purpose. You have learned what they needed to teach you so now you should feel free to release them, and to create in their place the life you have always dreamed of.

Finally, when your fire has burned out and the ashes have cooled, take the ashes and put them into the soil of a garden, a lawn, or of a potted plant. Let the ashes of something old and negative recycle into something new and positive.

THE GATEWAY MEDITATION

The Gateway Meditation is a twenty-minute exercise designed to help prepare you emotionally and spiritually for tomorrow's fast. It may seem simple, but it is actually a very effective process that will preview some of the issues that may surface for you during the fast. It will also help relax you. Try to do this meditation sometime before dinner on the last night of your prefast.

> To begin, you need to be in an area that is quiet and private. Your sacred space would be the ideal place. Relax in a comfortable chair, or sit comfortably on the floor cross-legged. Take a few deep breaths and slowly close your eyes.
>
> Imagine that you are about to embark on a very special journey that you have been looking forward to for a very long time. You have just arrived at the airport with everything you think you need to take with you on this trip. You have suitcases full of all of your favorite clothes and jewelry and mementos. You have your address book, your day-planner, your favorite magazines, your good luck charm, and lots of comfort foods for the trip. But just as you are boarding your flight, an announcement is made. You are told that the plane is carrying too much weight to take off safely, and that the only way you will be able to get to your destination is to shed everything you have brought with you. All of these things will be

stored safely, waiting for you when you return, but right now, you have to give up everything. No luggage, no carry-on items, no jewelry, no wallets, no anything.

What will you have to leave behind? Is it the cellular phone you were going to use to call your family? The expensive suits that help you cut your image in the world? The bottle of sleeping pills you take nightly? The candy bar in your pocket? Is it reams of work from the office? The beeper that keeps you always on call? The impressive gold watch that you never take off your wrist? The locket you wear around your neck? Your favorite photographs of your partner, your children, or your pets? The business cards with your prestigious job title? The keys to your car? The keys to your home? You may discover that some of the baggage you are being asked to leave behind has strong emotional components, perhaps even more powerful than you would have imagined.

If it helps, think of me as the person you are handing everything over to for safekeeping. I will help free you of all of those things you felt were absolutely necessary—things you felt you could not live without—and I will take good care of everything so you can get on that plane. I will treat these things with respect, with love, and with good care.

For the next fifteen minutes, try to imagine what it would be like to go on your journey free of everything you have brought with you. Not just physical objects, but emotional issues, pressures, and problems as well. For fifteen minutes, just let yourself float freely, unencumbered, alone.

For some of you, this will be very liberating. For some, it will be frightening. It may be the first time in your life that you have ever felt this way. The important thing is to hold on to this feeling for a full fifteen minutes. If you lose track of time, and are lucky enough to hold on to the feelings of freedom and weightlessness even longer, so much the better.

Now it is time to return. As I promised, I will be at the

gateway waiting for you and I will have everything you left behind. You can have it all back. But as you come through the gateway to reclaim what is yours, stop for a moment and think about what it is you are picking up. Think hard. Are they things that you still really want? Are they things that actually make you happy, or are they things you might want to leave behind during your days of fasting? Are you ready to shed these things the same way you will be shedding toxins and all of the other unhealthy and unwanted stuff that has been living in your body and affecting your well-being? When you have finished your meditation, it would be helpful to take a few minutes to write about this experience in your journal.

PLEASANT DREAMS

Before you go to bed tonight you might want to have a soothing cup of herbal tea. I find that chamomile tea is the best choice for this evening. Once you get into bed, I want you to do a simple breathing exercise:

THE CONNECTING BREATH

Lie on your back at first and gently place your palms on your stomach. Take a slow, deep breath. Feel the way your stomach expands as you breathe in. Now exhale slowly and fully. Feel the way your stomach contracts as you release the air you are holding inside you. Repeat this five more times—a deep inhale followed by a deep exhale—and be sure to do it slowly and purposefully each time, giving every breath meaning and power.

As you take these breaths, give your body a chance to let go of the memory of what you have been doing to it lately—the way you have been eating, the way you have been sleeping, and the way you have been taking care of yourself (or perhaps, to be more accurate, not taking care of yourself). These are all bad body memories, so you want to let them go. As you start to clear these memories out, you are opening the door for the good memory of well-being to come back into your cellular structure. You are going to be learning how to empty out the "bad" on all levels—physical, emotional, and spiritual—and it's important right now to start that by giving your body the message with your breath, with your thoughts, and with your feelings. So try to let it all go as you prepare to go to sleep. Let it all slip away, knowing that so much of your life is about to change.

PART THREE

THE 3-DAY ENERGY FAST

DAY 1 MENU

Hot Water and Lemon

MORNING DRINK	Pineapple-Papaya-Strawberry (pages 237–38)
MID-MORNING DRINK CHOICES	Apple-Strawberry-Grape Apple-Pear-Ginger (page 238)
LUNCH	Carrot-Beet-Apple (page 239)
AFTERNOON SNACK DRINK	Green Vegetable Drink (pages 239–40)
EVENING MEAL	Warm Vegetable Broth (pages 241–42)
DESSERT DRINK	See Choices (pages 242–43)

Water and herbal teas can be enjoyed throughout the day.

10

Day 1: Getting Still

I want you to love the experience of juice-fasting as much as I do, and I wish I could be there with each and every one of you during these three fasting days. No matter how many times I fast, either alone or with others, a three-day spiritual fast is always a wonderful adventure and a glorious journey. Enjoy it.

Day 1 is a day of change and new beginnings. Your diet, your actions, and your body are going to change today. Some of these changes will be temporary; some I hope you will choose to make permanent. Right now, the most important thing is that you invite all of these changes in and make them feel welcome.

I know you can make it through three days of juice-fasting. By Day 3, your own optimism and hopefulness will be transformed into a concrete sense of accomplishment, vitality, serenity, and well-being.

GOOD MORNING—TODAY YOU START BECOMING NEW

Before you do *anything* else this morning—before you go to the bathroom, brush your teeth, pet the dog, kiss your partner, or turn on CNN, you need to bring yourself into Day 1 with a loving welcome. It makes a big difference if you say it out loud, and say it as though you really mean it: "Good morning."

Welcome to this new day. Welcome to this process of growth and healing. Let yourself hear your own words, and let your body feel them fully. Greeting yourself is a way to remind yourself that today you and your inner world are *the* priorities. So even if it makes you feel a little self-conscious or slightly awkward, start the day by acknowledging the miracle of you, and your new healing agenda.

Your intention for today is to get calm and get still.

What does it mean to get still? I remember my reaction when I first heard the phrase. I thought to myself, "I'm already still. *Still* stressed, *still* confused, *still* driven." At the time, I thought that was pretty funny. Today, I'm not so sure.

Most of us spend our lives on the run. I even know people who eat their meals on wheels, having breakfast, lunch, and sometimes even dinner while driving in the car. Some men and women dress and primp behind the wheel while phoning and faxing on their cellular phones. Too many of us are racing to our appointments and racing *through* our appointments; we run to the gym, run in the gym, and run home from the gym. Even if we are sitting still, our minds are still racing: What do I need to do today? Where do I need to go? What will I wear? When will I eat? Who do I need to call? Do I have letters to write? Bills to pay? Will I get home in time for "Seinfeld"? Whew . . . Is this really living? Sure, you can get three thousand things done. And your days are full—jam-packed full. But more and more is feeling like less and less. That's why your intention for today is to get calm and get still.

IN ORDER TO START THE JOURNEY OF NEWNESS, WE STOP

Today you begin preparing for new life that's centered and balanced. That means creating space in your body and your psyche for all that is to come. This will happen naturally as you get calm and get still. So start by doing absolutely nothing—nothing but sitting quietly in bed and thinking about your intention for today. Right now, the tranquil state I have described might seem very foreign, yet it exists within you, as it exists within all of us.

Today's affirmation:
"Entering the stillness, I become new"

Repeat this affirmation out loud, under your breath, or think it. You can write it over and over again in your journal. Give yourself the opportunity and space right now to connect with this affirmation. Let the cadence of the words sink into your body, and let the meaning sink into your soul.

I like to have both an intention and an affirmation every day of the fast to give balance. The affirmation is the feminine, "yin" side of the process; it is the reassurance, the cradle, the warm blanket. The intention is the counterbalance, the masculine "yang"; it is the goal, the guiding principle, the clear shining light. Both affirmation and intention will guide you through the day. They will become your two hands, and you can call on either, depending on your needs.

BRUSHING AWAY THE OLD

Pick up your skin brush (it should be right by your bedside) and remember that you chose it with love to use with love. Start to brush your body, beginning with the soles of your feet. Brush in slow, firm, circular motions. Now work your way slowly up through both sides of the body, front and back. Go round and round on your calves, your knees, your thighs, your abdomen, your buttocks, your stomach, and up through your chest, *avoiding the breast area*. Continue around the back, the shoulders, the arms, and down the spine. Really allow yourself to explore your body surface with every movement of the brush. Notice the dips and shallows, the flats and the curves.

Every reinvigorating circular motion of your brush gives your body and your spirit a chance to let go of the memory of all of the toxic and negative things you have been holding on to. Let each circular motion of the brush against the body help you *realize* the patterns and interactions that have been draining you. Let go of all the ways in which you have not been healing and careful with your life. Let go of expectations, demands, failure scenarios as well as all the negative habits relating to eating, sleeping, and personal care. Brush away everything that has been making it impossible for you to accomplish your personal best. You want to *release* these obstructions from your life so you can *recharge* your life force.

As the old cells come off your skin, let the old memories start to come off with them. Let them go so you can make room for a new, recharged sense of well-being to sparkle from your system. *Realize, Release, Recharge*. Start to clear away the bad on every level so you can start to fill up with the good you have been holding within under lock and key. Take your time. You want to really give your circulation a wake-up. Some people brush for five full minutes, others brush for forty-five minutes. Don't look at a clock. Let the process speak to you and do what feels best. Give your body a deep, caring massage, while giving your spirit a message of love and hope. When you're finished, stop for a moment and relax. Feel how every pore of your skin is alive and open to the day.

THE FIRST DRINK OF THE DAY: LEMON AND HOT WATER FOR PURIFYING

I like to put a slice of lemon in the cup first, so that the hot water is instantly infused with the essence of the lemon the moment it makes contact. Hot water with lemon is a great way to begin the cleansing and purification process; the bite of the fresh lemon will also help wake you up as the steam from the water rises to caress your face. Sip, and sip slowly.

CLEANSE AND DETOX IN THE MORNING BATH

You want the water for your morning bath to be warm, but not scalding hot. Choose from your selection of bath salts and pour at least one full handful into the bath. Enter the bath, and try to fully relax. Let the warmth penetrate down through your skin, deeper and deeper to your body's core. Look at your body with kindness as you soak. Ask the water to come into your pores and help you become new. Let it carry away all the noise and confusion in your life. Feel the buoyancy and the healing.

If you really can't adjust to a bath, it's okay to shower, but make it a luxurious shower. Try to imagine that you're standing under a glorious waterfall or that you're on a tropical island surrounded by flowers and a fragrant breeze. Give the water a chance to soak into your skin.

There are no rules about time here. When you want to get out of the tub, don't reach for perfumes or colognes. Instead, try a few dots of essential rosemary oil on your wrists, your neck, or behind your ears.

YOUR MORNING MEDITATION AND BREATH WORK

To do this meditation properly you need to be wearing comfortable, loose-fitting clothing. You don't want any part of your body to feel constricted. Go to your sacred space and sit cross-legged on the floor. Sit on a small pillow so that you are leaning slightly forward. This will stop your legs from falling asleep, and it will also increase your comfort. You can also sit against a wall to straighten your back more easily; it is very important that your spine is straight, particularly during the breathing exercises. This way of sitting may seem slightly awkward in the beginning, but you will become comfortable with this new configuration over the next three days.

Lock your buttocks together against the ground and straighten out your spine, imagining that you are letting it flow up along a tall silk thread that pulls up, up, and out the top of your head. Find the rhythm of your breath. Now slow your breathing down a fraction and then take five deep breaths, one after the other. With each breath, imagine that a giant vacuum is coming inside of you to vacuum up all of the old internal stuff you want to get rid of. Each time you take a breath, allow your mind to relax and your body to settle, keeping it open to all sensations. Within the physical surroundings of your sacred space, you are entering into your *internal* sacred space. There, stop for a moment, and remember that breath is life, breath gives life, and breath is our constant reminder that we are alive. Then go on to today's first breathing exercise:

ALTERNATE NOSTRIL BREATHING

Keeping your mouth closed, press your right nostril closed with the thumb of your right hand and breathe in slowly through your left nostril. Now close your left nostril with the ring finger from your right hand, and hold both nostrils closed for a moment. Release the pressure on your right nostril, and breathe out slowly through your right nostril. Bring the air back in through your right nostril, keeping the left nostril closed with your ring finger. Close both nostrils for a moment, then open your left nostril and slowly let the air out again. It's like you're creating a little cavity of air in your nose, letting it go up to your third eye, and then out again through the opposite nostril.

Alternate Nostril Breathing balances the mind, keeping it quiet and disengaged from the thoughts that may be trying to get your attention and distract you. If you do have thoughts, don't get anxious, and don't actively try to push them away. Let them dance across your consciousness until they drift out and away. Continue with your Alternate Nostril Breathing. Within a minute or two, your body will let you know that it is time to stop. At this point, bring both palms to rest lightly on both knees for a moment, sensing you have already cast away a layer of tension. Rest quietly for a minute or two before moving on to your morning meditation.

The Golden Guided Meditation

Imagine a little golden ball, a ball of sunshine, positioned in the center of your stomach. Before you start to play with it, just look at it. Imagine that this ball is filled with a beautiful golden liquid, a gel-like liquid. It's very warm. Not hot, but just the right temperature, like perfectly warmed honey.

Let the ball fall to the very bottom of one foot and let it rest there. Now let it slowly move through the sole of your foot, from toe to toe, and back to your ankle and up your leg. Once it reaches the top of your leg, let it slip down the other leg and repeat its journey up until it starts moving through your body. As it moves, feel it nourishing every cell that it passes, while it also pulls from those same cells all the toxins that have been hiding or lingering for years and years.

Allow the golden ball to absorb the old aches and pains, the bad memories of past experiences that settle and reside in the muscles and tissues of the body. Allow your toxicities—the anger, the emotional states you can't control, the compulsive behaviors, the snacks and unhealthy foods, the many medications—to be sponged up and removed into the warmth of the golden ball.

Sense the ball as it travels. Up through your shins, through your calves, along your legs, through every inch of your musculature, and through every bone. Feel it moving through your tissues and through your bloodstream. Wherever the ball travels, feel it bring you new strength. Now allow the ball to move up through your knees, through your thighs and up into the groin and abdomen where it expands to fill, cleanse, and energize you. Feel the sexual parts of you being replenished and invigorated. Feel your belly full, and feel the aliveness in your energy center, the center of your stomach, the place that gives so many of us trouble because it is where we store our grief, our anger, our anxieties, and our pain. Let it heal your digestive system, and let the golden gel replenish the personal power you have in life like a refreshed memory. Let the ball rest here for a few moments. Breathe fully and deeply—breaths that make full use of the body. Feel your strength. Feel your center.

Let the ball move again. Let it move up through the belly and into the chest, around the heart. Allow the golden liquid to bathe your heart in loving support. Find the places where your heart needs comforting and mending, and let it cradle and soothe you with warmth, kindness, and peacefulness; let it fill you with emotional encouragement, trust, and hope. Let your cells absorb this into their memory as the golden ball fills you and feeds you with everything you deserve.

Allow the golden liquid to come up through your shoulders. Let it relax you, relieving the emotional and spiritual burdens you carry. Let it move like a deep heating massage through your shoulders, down through your arms into your hands, and through your fingers to all that you have touched. Let yourself remember all the things you have touched and feel your memories as sacred, as knowledge, as wisdom.

Now bring the ball back up through the arms and shoulders until it is poised at the base of your neck, at the very top of your spine. Slowly, let the ball drop down through the length of your spine, making every inch of your spinal cord shiny and new. When it reaches the bottom, bring it back up through the spine and into the back of your throat. In your throat, let the ball swallow all of the words that you have said, all the words that you are not saying, and clear the throat chakra, the channel through which you express yourself to the world. Swallow fully and feel it clear.

Nearing the end of the meditation, allow the liquid now to come up through the sinuses, melting down any obstacles, any passages that are blocked. Use every breath to clear your nostrils, up and around into the passages behind your eyes. As you do this, wipe clear the vision of all that you have seen. Let the golden gel absorb and carry off anything that has been painful to witness.

Let the warmth now flow through your ears, melting away the words that still ring inside your head. Let it remove all the harsh, unkind, thoughtless words you have heard others say, or heard yourself speak; all that you have agreed with, not agreed with, or not heard enough of, or that has been too loud. Feel your ears cleansed.

Finally let the liquid gel expand and fill your entire head with its cleansing warmth. Let it absorb the patterns of behavior, the habits, and the obstacles to healthy change. Release yourself into the powerful and kind warmth, letting your brain soak in this healing bath.

Sink into yourself. Feel all the new cells breathing in your body, the power of your flowing blood, the raw strength of your bones, and the formation of new muscle. Come into the stillness of your own power. Embrace all that is inside you, and know that it is sacred.

Let your breath connect you back into your physical body. Coming out of the meditation, as if you were coming out of a gorgeous, restful sleep, take a couple of deep luscious breaths. From your toes to your head, connect with your power, your unique voice and vision, and, most essentially, connect with your heart. Your refreshed physical being is already connecting to your intention, to get calm and get still. Remember today's affirmation, and say it to yourself now: "Entering the stillness, I become new."

INDULGING IN YOUR MORNING DRINK

PINEAPPLE-PAPAYA-STRAWBERRY (pages 237–38)

What a welcoming sight awaits you in the kitchen this morning. This is the payoff for your hours of preparation, a lovely space stocked with everything you need to make your juice for the next three days. As you prepare your drinks today, you might want to say a little blessing, or you can just glory in the beauty of the colors and textures of your produce.

Take the glass you selected for yourself and pour it to the brim with your fabulous morning drink. Take it to the table you set so beautifully last night, sit down comfortably, and pause for a moment. It is time to have your drink. Take your first mouthful and chew it slowly in your mouth. That's right—chew it as though it were solid food. Feel it on your tongue, against the walls of your mouth, between your teeth. Do nothing but focus on your drink. Don't read the newspaper, don't turn on the radio, and don't turn on the TV. Stay in your chair and stay focused on your drink. As you slowly chew each mouthful, notice how rich the experience of a simple drink can be, and how good that feels. As you taste the wonderful sweetness, repeat your affirmation: "Entering the stillness, I become new."

MORNING ENERGY WORK

1: AND NOW A WORD FROM MOTHER NATURE

As you head outside for a beautiful nature walk, try to imagine that a wonderful wise spiritual guide is walking with you helping you notice things that you've never noticed before. Maybe if it feels good, you'll want to walk for an hour or even longer. Try the Walking Meditation on page 93.

2: FINDING YOUR OWN VOICE

Starting a new life begins by saying "No" to the life you have right now. It means crying out till all that is good in the universe hears you and rushes in to meet your needs. So follow the instructions on pages 94–96 and start practicing those "Nos."

You may want to scream into a pillow, muffle your screams with background music, scream in the shower, or scream in your car. Or you might prefer an outdoor spot (a deserted beach, the woods, or a park) if that gives you a forum where you know you can get really loud without feeling self-conscious because there is no one around to hear you. I usually do this on the beach, screaming out into the sea. I get really loud. This is not a time for gentility or softness. Let it out! Clean out those pipes! After ten or fifteen minutes of this releasing exercise, give yourself a few extra minutes to reconnect with and refocus on today's intention.

THE MID-MORNING DRINK

The Mid-Morning Drink is a refreshing pick-me-up after your spirited but intense energy work. Your choices are:

Apple-Strawberry-Grape
Apple-Pear-Ginger
(recipes page 238)

DAY 1: MORNING JOURNAL-WRITING—GETTING RID OF THE OLD

The morning of Day 1 is a beautiful time to start writing down all the negative things you want to remove from your life, and all the positive things you want to add. When you write to detoxify from the negative baggage you have been carrying, you may find your words reflecting intense emotions you have locked away. Don't be critical about your negative feelings. Just write and let them out. Write about the patterns you've been locked into, the people you've put up with, the disappointments you've felt, the "shoulds," the "musts," and the "better off ifs."

Write any way you like on the page—up and down, big or small, in black and white or in colors. Find and follow your own yellow brick road. Don't worry about posterity or penmanship. Focus on connecting paper, ink (or pencil), and your heart.

LATE-MORNING YOGA

Relax and surrender yourself to the experience of yoga. As you do these exercises (see pages 221–36), gently try to experience in your body an awareness of places that have become stagnant, and places that feel dark, or filled with emotions. Your yoga movements will help you break up and move these old emotional centers, giving you the chance to experience a true, clearer center.

Notice how different your breath feels after you have finished the yoga. Comfortable. Friendly. Before you move on to the Lunch Drink, take some time to do a few of the Connecting Breaths you experienced for the first time the night before the fast. Let yourself fully feel each vital breath in the stomach. Inhale, stomach out. Exhale, stomach in. Really use your nostrils. Remember to hold each breath for seven counts. Don't rush. Relax. With each cycle, you can feel the edges of stillness around and inside you.

LET'S DO LUNCH

CARROT-BEET-APPLE (recipe page 239)

This juice gives new meaning to the expression "power lunch." I love this drink because after the cleansing morning fruit beverages you can feel the different energy of this combination. It's so explosive and revitalizing that there is almost an electric sizzle to it.

This lunch drink is a terrific liver "mover." The liver is where most toxins are metabolized, and it's particularly important to keep this organ revitalized during your fast. While Carrot-Beet-Apple is a great drink for fasting, it is also a wonderful drink to have as a regular part of your food regime to energize your liver and its vital functions.

Use this time to reconnect again with today's intention to get calm and get still. As you slowly sip your juice, try to be conscious of everything you are doing and everything that is happening around you. The sound of any music you may be playing, the vibrant color of the drink, and the stillness that is growing around you.

Do you feel as though you are moving in some strange slow motion? That suggests that you've been doing many things way too fast. People always tell you that "less is more," but they never seem to tell you what that means. It's hard to "take time to stop and smell the roses," when your life is moving so fast you don't even *see* the rosebush. But that is really what life is all about, and you need to discover this now, not thirty years from now when all you can do is mourn for what you have missed. So let yourself appreciate today's lunch juice, and the lessons that it offers. Not only will this meal become unforgettable, but hopefully, it will mark the beginning of a more complete, "digested" way of living.

AN AFTERNOON OF CHANGE

As you move into the afternoon on your first day, you may feel yourself getting restless or edgy. You might think that the way to combat these uncomfortable feelings is to run a mile, make a thousand phone calls, whirl like a dervish, or clean, dust, and vacuum every room of your home. Yet what you really need to do is go deeper into a relaxing, soothing space.

You are at your first breakthrough point in the purifying process. Now, more than ever, you don't want to turn away from the portal, but to walk through, bravely. If you're not sure you can do this alone, visualize your Gatekeeper alongside of you and let his/her support, encouragement, and wisdom give you strength and faith.

CREATING COMFORT: FINDING PEACE IN SILENT ACTIVITIES

Those of you who went to summer camp may remember "free periods," those times when you got to choose what you wanted to do from a list of specific activities. This is one of those "free periods." Silence will enhance or become your free time. You be the judge.

Select an activity that is best for the needs of your body and spirit. If you feel tired, give yourself permission to close your eyes or take a nap. You might enjoy taking a soothing bath, or savoring a cup of herbal tea while listening to some of the music you selected to accompany you on the fast. Consider doing a slow breathing exercise. Choose from:

Connecting Breath (page 120)

Alternate Nostril Breathing (page 130)

Meditation is another excellent choice at this point in the day. You may want to repeat one of the meditations you have learned already, or even make up your own.

In this place of meditation and dedication, ask the mind to join you in the most still part of yourself, the most beautiful, enriching part of your soul that is giving you the gift of this fast. Let yourself connect to the deepest parts of you that gave you the idea to seek balance and detox, and the encouragement and energy to make it through. Complimenting yourself in this way makes you feel loved and alive because it acknowledges the soul's purpose to be calm, clear, and clean.

Remember that spiritual book you have been waiting to read? Now would be a wonderful time to open it. *Care of the Soul, The Way of the Peaceful Warrior,* or some wonderful poetry by Rumi. This is an ideal time to relax and connect with the inspiration that can be found in a book devoted to the spirit. Try to stay away from the kind of reading that brings you back into the freneticism of the day-to-day world.

DON'T FORGET YOUR JOURNAL

If you don't feel in the mood to write very much, at least do a five-minute journal "check-in." Basically, that means opening your journal and writing one or two sentences about where you are emotionally, physically, and spiritually at this particular point in the fast. For example: "Day 1. Just had lunch drink. Feeling jittery, uncertain." Or "Day 1. Just had lunch drink. Feeling fabulous, already different."

Treat your afternoon like a "happy hour." Not a time to sip screwdrivers or eat peanuts, but a time to do something that makes you *truly* happy. This is a great "try time"—a time to try something new you have always promised yourself, or something old you need to reconnect with. Maybe take out some paper and pastels; perhaps you prefer modeling clay. I recommend finger painting to those who resist thinking of themselves as artistic. Let yourself have the kind of fun a small child can have when he or she gets lost in a world of colors and textures.

Spend these afternoon hours getting still and replenishing your energy. Drink as much water or herbal tea as you like and as often as you like. Keeping yourself hydrated will fend off lightheadedness and headaches, and the act of continually sipping *something*—even if it's only water—will ward off the feeling of being deprived or tortured.

One final thought before you finish your energy-replenishing afternoon. I would like you to clasp your hands together firmly in a shake, then put your arms around yourself and give yourself a sincere, big hug. Be proud. Shower yourself with compliments. You have just come through one of the most challenging parts of Day 1, and you have succeeded with flying colors. Now you can celebrate, and refresh yourself with an Afternoon Snack Drink.

AFTERNOON SNACK DRINK

GREEN VEGETABLE DRINK (pages 239–40)

The purifying strategy you are practicing involves cleansing fruit juices in the morning, rebuilding vegetable juices in the afternoon, and a balancing broth in the evening. You will be having this delicious green vegetable drink to oxygenate and purify your system every day of your fast.

PREPARING YOUR EVENING MEAL

WARM VEGETABLE BROTH (page 241)

Tonight, and every night of the fast, the main event is this warm, stunning vegetable broth. The broth is rich in potassium, and that makes it a great "balancer" at the end of each inspiring, yet draining (if not exhausting) day. Make enough broth tonight to last for all three evenings of the fast. For those of you who are integrating Day 2 and Day 3 of fasting into a back-to-work schedule, this will be particularly useful, but it is my experience that most people are grateful that they have less work to do on the evenings of Day 2 and Day 3.

Don't get caught up in a maddening frenzy of slicing and dicing. Keep your movements slow and deliberate and stay focused on the pleasure of the process and the promise of health and wholeness. Listen to some music while you cook, or do some vocalization exercises in the kitchen.

EVENING BREATHING TRANSITION

Time for the 5 o'clock news? Not today. On this first day of your fast, you make the transition from the afternoon into the evening by practicing Push Breathing. Today, what's "out there" is not important. You need to stay with what's inside.

PUSH BREATHING—THE ROAD BACK HOME

Of all the breathing exercises, I feel this is the great cleanser. Not only does it relieve anxiety and stress, it relaxes the facial muscles, tones the skin around your eyes, and eases the lines of discontent around your mouth. Push Breathing is a spa in itself—a minivacation without the travel. Here's how it's done.

> Open your mouth wide, really wide. Now take your tongue and push it all the way out, as if you were trying to reach across the room with it. Like a lion, say HHAAAHH! And again HHAAAHH! And again HHAAAHH! Let this sound come from the back of your throat, clearing all the words out of your being. Push out resentment, spite, sadness, and any second thoughts you are harboring back there. Push out depression, anxiety, and disappointments. Let all that negativity out with a rush! HHAAAHH! Keep saying it with your tongue way out there, as far and as wide as it can go. And don't be intimidated by your own power. If this exercise makes you feel self-conscious, muffle your sounds with background music.

Prepare to be surprised by the force of the sound that comes out of you. We hold so much negative emotion deep inside ourselves because of our emotional commitment to not saying what we really want or need to say. There are *so* many toxic pockets in each of us. But you are turning all this negativity away from you now. And it's about time. So take that debris and . . . push! Confront it and release it so you can get on with the positive growth in your life.

Push Breathing is also a terrific toner for those times when you have pushed your body and mind too far—done too many activities, tried to meet too many demands, had a serious argument, started to feel sick, etc. In times of great stress, this clearing breath de-stresses the body and brings you back to your very own center.

CREATE A MAGICAL MOOD FOR DINNER

Dinner should be a special time. Create a dinner setting for yourself at the table using linens, candles, flowers . . . the works. Of course, put out the special bowl and spoon you have chosen to use tonight—I use my best china and silver, and it completely elevates me. If it suits your mood, put on music. If the weather permits, and you desire it, dine alfresco.

I think it's very important to dress up for dinner—nothing uncomfortable or constraining, but definitely a little more elegant than your standard daytime clothing. If you have something made of silk, indulge. Men shouldn't try to wear neckties, but a sport jacket definitely adds an element of elegance that you deserve to share with yourself.

If your family is eating with you tonight, encourage everyone to dress up and surrender to the magic. You want the others to join you in your celebration, not tease you for trying something new and different. Don't keep them in the dark. On the contrary, talk to them about your day and let them ask you questions. Ask them to try their hardest to remain calm and gentle around you. You are in the cocoon stages of your new being right now, and you need to be addressed and related to with great understanding, sensitivity, and care. It's okay to express your vulnerability, even if they think you're the Rock of Gibraltar.

NURTURING YOURSELF—ONE SPOONFUL AT A TIME

Ladle your broth into your waiting bowl (or bowls, if others are joining you) and then sit down to the balancing meal you deserve. I like to say a word of blessing before I start to sip my broth. This blessing is nothing more than a few simple words of thanks for the wonderful day that the universe has allowed me to have. Simple words, yes, but important ones nonetheless. Perhaps you already have a blessing that you use at special mealtimes. If you don't, take the time to say *something* that sincerely acknowledges this meal and this day. If you're not accustomed to doing this, it may seem awkward, but that feeling will pass, and the connection you have made to a larger picture will remain to ground you and remind you how very special all of life's moments should be.

As you look at the bowl of warm broth in front of you, you might be feeling incredibly grateful. On the other hand, you could be thinking, "Oh my God, is this it???" Yes, this *is* it, but prepare to be surprised by how full your stomach feels by the time you have finished *slowly* sipping as much of this nourishing broth as you want. Relax as the warm, nutrient-rich liquid soothes and expands your stomach. The next question is, will you feel truly satisfied? Frankly, it would be unfair for me to promise that you will.

It's only Day 1, and that means that neither your body nor your psyche has probably made enough of a transition to feel *completely* satisfied right now by a few bowls of warm broth. You need to remind yourself that you're just at the beginning stages. You might be thinking about that cheeseburger again. That's okay. Thinking about cheeseburgers isn't breaking the law. But try to stay in the moment and focus on your goals to Cleanse, Rebuild, and Balance. You have already accomplished so much. Try to make this a gratifying meal in a peaceful moment. And let yourself be happy at the stillness you are allowing into your life. If it's possible, try to have your meal in silence. You have the company of your food.

As you finish your dinner, you might feel a slight shiver of anticipation about tomorrow. After all, this evening is coming to an end, but there are still two full days that lie ahead of you. Try to avoid projecting into the future at this point. You are doing just fine right now, and that is important. You will work through Day 2 and Day 3 when they arrive.

When you have finished your broth, take a few minutes to sit in your sacred space and let your dinner work quietly to balance your system. Put your hands on your full stomach and breathe quietly, slowly, and deeply.

THE DESSERT DRINK

Some of you will feel too full to put another drop of anything into your stomach; you may even have trouble finishing a single bowl of broth. But if you're not one of those people and still have room in your tummy for something extra, take a look at the dessert juices on pages 242–43.

EVENING COMFORTS BEFORE BED

Take a warm bath before going to bed tonight. This is a comforting cleaning after a long day of detoxing. Use your bath salts and aromatherapy oils; hops or sandalwood oil will really help you relax. Set a calming mood for yourself with gentle music and special lighting. Candles would be great tonight—I love to soak in the tub and get lost in the hypnotic flickering of candlelight. You may want to play with some of your bath toys too. Or you may just want to close your eyes and let the various scents and sensations consume you.

MIRROR, MIRROR— ARE YOU TALKING TO ME?

I want you to spend some time in front of the mirror before you go to bed. You need to visually connect to your body this evening—even if it feels a little awkward—in order to fully appreciate the nuances of transformation that are already visible. When you have dried off from your bath, stand in front of a large mirror, preferably a full-length mirror, and take a good long look at yourself. As you look at yourself in the mirror, congratulate yourself on already getting through the most difficult parts of this day. Tell yourself it was a breeze. Let yourself feel your strength. Tell yourself that you are beautiful, handsome, gorgeous, spectacular, fabulous, and fantastic. And try to say it like you mean it, because the truth is that you really are.

Before retiring, why not indulge in a delicious cup of herbal tea? There are so many great choices—chamomile, dandelion, licorice, spearmint, and Sleepy Time, to mention a few. Stay away from activating teas like peppermint and ginger; they are better to drink earlier in the day. Add a sliver of lemon. Sip slowly, and enjoy the tranquillity of this moment.

TUCK YOURSELF IN WITH YOUR BEST FRIEND —YOUR JOURNAL

Use your journal to retrace everything you want to let go of emotionally, physically, and spiritually. Write about everything you want to leave you; all the things you are ready to say good-bye to. Write as much as you can. Unleash yourself and unburden yourself. The more you "empty out" your mind before bed, the more fully you will be able to rest tonight.

Before you go to bed, here's one last exercise. Make a list of all the habits, compulsions, and self-destructive behavior patterns that are no longer serving you. Write this list on a little piece of paper. Turn this list into a dream bundle by crumpling it up and putting it under your pillow. As you turn out the lights and put your head on the pillow, ask to be released from all of these behavior patterns that are no longer serving you. In the morning, throw your little "bundle" away.

PERCHANCE TO DREAM . . .

As you lie in bed and close your eyes, connect one last time with today's intention. Think about what your goal was for today—to get calm and get still. Think about all of the ways in which you accomplished that goal. Now think about today's affirmation, and whisper the words to yourself as a good-night blessing: "In the stillness, I become new."

Close your eyes, place your hands on your stomach, and breathe deeply. Breathe yourself free of the past, and into sleep. You are well on your way to unburdening yourself of so much that no longer serves you, or has never served you well. Welcome sleep into your new-opportunity mind. Welcome sleep into your body that is regenerating itself into healthy meridian alignment. Welcome the silence; welcome the peacefulness; welcome the night.

If, by any chance, you get up in the middle of the night for a bathroom break, and you are tempted by the thought of food, you should have some snack juice left over in the refrigerator.

DAY 2 MENU

Hot Water and Lemon

MORNING DRINK	Pineapple-Papaya-Strawberry (pages 237–38)
MID-MORNING DRINK CHOICES	Pineapple-Pear-Lemon Grape (pages 240 and 239)
LUNCH	Carrot-Cabbage-Apple (page 241)
AFTERNOON SNACK DRINK	Green Vegetable Drink (pages 239–40)
EVENING MEAL	Warm Vegetable Broth (page 241–42)
DESSERT DRINK	See Choices (pages 242–43)

Water and herbal teas can be enjoyed throughout the day.

11

Day 2: Finding Faith

Fasten your seat belt. It's Day 2, and almost everyone feels that Day 2 is the hardest day. Although today may start out as a day of doubt, it will turn into a day of faith because today you are going to discover that there is a source deep within you that can take you anywhere you want to go.

A SPECIAL MORNING

Do you have any morning rituals? Things you do or think as you move from dreams to consciousness? I do. I sing to my dog, who runs into my bedroom every morning thrilled with the new day and the wonder of being alive. A person might wake up thinking, "Oh God, it's Monday." My dog never feels that way. Her favorite song is "Some Enchanted Evening," which I change to doggy language for her: lots of barks, yelps, and howls. I also use this morning time to teach her how to do "paws-on healing." Obviously, my ritual is about making a connection. Not everyone has a pet, but we can all have rituals to help us move into the day with a sense of joy.

Today is a good day to establish or strengthen the connecting rituals in your life. As you are lying in bed, take some time to really give thanks for your being, your family, and your life. Let yourself consciously acknowledge the specialness of this day, your existence, and everything and everyone that supports you. Because of all these things, you have made it to this day, and you will make it through this day.

To help get moving, try this little exercise for *Good Energy*.

> Start by taking your palms and rubbing them together to create friction and heat. Then gently slap the bottom of your soles with your warm palms and wake them up. Take your hands and slap up and down the sides of your legs, all the way up your thighs. Be gentle: *no hitting allowed!* You are waking up the *chi*—the energy and vital force—in your body. Slap up and down your arms. Then slap the base of your spine and the top of your spine, moving morning energy into the cells. If your hands lose their energy, rub them together again. Finally, put your energized hands over your eyes to clear up morning fogginess.

A DAY OF OPPORTUNITIES

Day 1 was a "day of changes," a day of settling down. But today, Day 2, is a "day of opportunities," a day of stirring it up. Although this will be your breakthrough day, you need to be prepared to feel colossally daunted, as many obstacles will typically appear in your path to test your commitment and test your resolve. There may be times that you feel like you are climbing Mount Everest—in flip-flops, no less. Your body and mind may experience enormous pressure. Or you might resonate with such a kaleidoscope of emotions you could swear that you were channeling the sixties. This is how just a few people have expressed their experience of Day 2.

I am telling you this not to discourage you, only to prepare you. With preparation, Day 2 is nothing more than a day of challenges that provide splendid opportunities. Today, for example, you will probably be grateful that you asked your family and friends to give you the space you needed to detox as healing crises introduce themselves: mild dizziness, slight nausea, headaches, itchiness, hot and cold flashes, tenderness of the skin, constipation, flatulence, fatigue, achiness, and all-around crankiness. Not fun, I know, but these are important signs that your body is getting its act together so it can take you down a new road. Movement is going from in to out as toxins exit your body.

Throughout the day, conflicted dialogues may well dance in your head. "Even if I know that elements of my life are toxic, I'm still going to have to go back to it in three days . . . so what's the point?" "I have all these goals, or I think I do . . . do I? Or am I just kidding myself?" You start thinking in "maybe" language. "Maybe this fast would be better to do some other time." "Maybe there's something else that would work better, or faster, or more easily." "Maybe if I stopped right now, I would already have the benefits I really needed." "Maybe this is the craziest thing I have ever tried to do." "No one can live on a juice island!"

No indeed. No one can. And no one is asking you to. Three days is not a lifetime, *it's only three days*. I call all those clamoring voices in your head "The Committee." These are the same voices that put all the "shoulds" in your life: you *should* do this; you *should* do that. These voices represent "toxic reasoning," and these are the voices that keep you from connecting with and following your deepest, most profound, most beautiful, and most powerful self. So for today, give The Committee a day off—let them go take a meeting on their own.

FIRST YOU CHANGE

That's what I tell people who are beginning to wonder whether the fasting ritual can make a difference in their lives.

Because you and your cells really are changing, this may be a turbulent day. It may even be a harrowing day. But *you will be okay*. I can say this because I have sat through this day with hundreds of people, and spoken about it with many hundreds more. And I can say it because I have been through this day myself over and over and over and over, each time victorious. I know how much work you did to bring yourself to this point, and I know that throughout this day you will be able to handle your doubts and fears.

THEN YOUR LIFE CHANGES

One of the by-products of getting centered is coming into a genuine state of consciousness. You have already arrived at a still point and it should be easier for you to see the madness that is swirling around you. You are going through this process so you can see things with a greater clarity, and get to the real heart of the issues in your life. And that's what is happening. Today your questions are becoming more focused and honed. You may unsettle yourself, but you will not unbalance yourself. You may feel as though you are spinning, but your center will hold because you gave it to yourself yesterday. That's what all that work was about. And this is the payoff.

You will probably find that this new clarity is giving you a greater sense of purpose. You are beginning to see down the road of your life, and are beginning to ask yourself larger questions in your life such as, "What is the path I need to follow?" Conflicting thoughts may be competing for space in your head. One minute you may be thinking about your purpose in life, and the next minute all you can think about is the ever-pressing question: "When will this day be over?" When all these conflicting thoughts find a way to coexist in our heads, then we become calm.

To find your spirit, and to find and hold on to your correct path, requires real faith. And that brings us to today's intention.

Your intention for today is to find faith—
to learn to stand back from your life
and let it evolve as it was meant to be.

I tell each person to imagine that he or she is on top of a lovely wave. It may be a little scary, but stay still and balanced and just ride it out. That's how you will make it to shore. When you do, you are going to feel exhilarated and wonderful—like someone who just rode a wave to the shore. So don't run away. Now, more than ever before, you need to trust the process of the fast. How will you find this faith? Believe it or not, if you hold your center, and stay with the program throughout this day, faith will find you.

It's easy for me to say "trust the process" because I've already lived through it many times. But this process is still a stranger to you. I recognize that it takes great strength and faith to let this stranger into your life and believe that it won't hurt you. Most of us have a lifetime of reasons to not trust *anything*. We have lost faith in society, we have lost faith in religion, we have lost faith in medicine, we have lost faith in "experts," and we have lost faith in ourselves. All of this will challenge you on Day 2.

Finding faith means more than just finding faith in the cleansing process and your ability to see this day through. It also means allowing yourself to become vulnerable and trusting about your place in the universe. You know that joke: How do you make God laugh?—Tell him your plans. This speaks to me because faith and trust are major issues in my life. We all need to better learn how to let go and stop trying to control our lives and everything that happens in them. Today, you will take giant steps toward releasing your need to control. One of the reasons we lose faith is because we try to control everything. When you feel as though everything rests with you, how can you find the bigger picture?

As you release control, try to see how this step helps you fill your life with new possibilities. As you and your cells change, begin to release the old and invite in the new. Trust your life to work in the best way possible. I know this to be true, but I am only your coach. If you are to fully realign your own spiritual spine, this faith and conviction must ultimately come from you.

You came to this process because you knew on some level, or on many levels, that with each passing year of your life you were abandoning the real person that you are and the life that you could be living. And you wanted desperately to repair that gap, before it was too late.

Now, you really *are* riding a wave, and a wave is not empty, it is strong and solid. You have the support of everything around you that is sound, and it will keep you buoyed and keep you strong. Today, you are being carried by the forces of positive direction and honest spirit. You will not sink, and you will not drown. You will navigate ably and proudly and beautifully. And by the end of this day, you may even feel yourself soar.

Today's affirmation: "I surrender to the bigger picture."

Today's affirmation is about releasing and permitting about letting down resistance. Say it to yourself right now, say it aloud, and be sure to keep saying it—as often as you wish—throughout this day.

On this day of finding faith, open up all the doors in your life. This is the part of my life where I allow spiritual guides to help me. We all have spiritual guides, no matter what we call them. Frequently spiritual guides enter our lives in the form of time and place. We are standing on a specific place at a specific moment—if we let go of control, we let possibility into our lives. Let go, and acknowledge that there is power in this world that is much larger and wiser than you, and you allow the pure energy of that greater power to connect with your center and your inner world. This simple intention invites unlimited possibility. By letting yourself be open and humble, you are actually setting the stage for magic.

I know what it feels like when you try to force the world to give you what you think you need. I also know that it doesn't work. We fight for control all of the time. From the smallest things like parking spaces and second helpings, to bigger issues like job direction and relationship growth. But the truth is that it just doesn't work. Control can only come from letting go of control, from surrendering to what is not "I-centered," and agreeing that things will happen that none of us can predict or imagine, let alone mastermind.

I like to think of this as higher learning—experiencing something above you and around you that is bigger than just you. Fear and the need to control keeps us spiritually toxic. Surrender, and a thousand-pound weight will be lifted from your shoulders. Invite the universe in, and you will truly become free.

I would like to say a few words here about patience. It's been very difficult for me to learn patience because I have to work against a tendency to push. I've had to learn to stay centered and take each of life's curves very, very slowly, letting things evolve as they were meant to be. My lesson has been to do one thing at a time, to do it well, and to let go of the outcome.

Let today's affirmation reassure you that you are not an isolated point, spinning with no rhyme or reason. You are not alone. You have the force of something cosmically powerful shoring you up. This larger force may not yet be apparent to you, but it is there and you are linked to it. Savor this affirmation. Let it cradle you, softening your anxieties and quieting your fears.

TREAT YOURSELF WITH KINDNESS

Think of yourself as a young, tender being, and give yourself unconditional acceptance. Accept that what you are doing with this cleanse is not only good, but wonderful. And just do the best you can. If you feel like you did a better job or had a better attitude yesterday on Day 1, don't get worried. Expect a little bit of anxiety, but don't let it get the better of you. You may find that as you cleanse, the worry will ooze out of your system, like perspiration dripping off you after good workout. So go ahead and get that worry out!

If you have schedules and life demands that *must* be attended to, don't panic. Just, as they say, do it. Walk the dog, make that presentation, pick your child up from school, and don't concern yourself with possible consequences. You are not undoing your detox process. Your cleansing is ongoing, even though it may not be in first gear while you are getting these other activities accomplished. Try to be very Zen about what you're doing—become the motion.

Throughout this day, just put your intention and affirmation in front of you always, and surround them with light at the third eye, at the center of your forehead, and take a moment to meditate wherever you can. This will carry you through the day and your center will hold.

STARTING THIS DAY

While you are still in bed, begin the day with five deep Connecting Breaths. Place the palms of your hands on your stomach and do five of the deep inhales/exhales you have been practicing for the past two days. Inhale, stomach out. Exhale, stomach in. Let the pattern of your breath be your only thought. This is the fastest, most effective way to get centered. Use your breath to help prepare you for today.

Follow the same routine as you did yesterday:

- *A refreshing cup of hot water and lemon*
  As you sip, think about your many fortunes and open the door to the possibilities of this new day. Think about the miracle that is you. Think about the power and genius that was involved in creating you, and remember that this day is about connecting with the divine that resides in you.
- *A thorough skin-brushing*
  Treat yourself like a garden that needs gentle tending. As you gently brush in a circular motion, you are removing debris to allow new healthy shoots to grow toward the sun. Brush the nooks and crannies—the sensitive areas behind your knees, and the neglected areas in the small of your back. Allow the action of today's brushing to remove all remainders of yesterday. Brush away yesterday's thoughts, moods, and struggles. *Realize, Release, Recharge.* Bring yourself into a tingling present awareness of *Today*.
- *A healing morning bath*
  You want those toxins you are releasing from their ancient resting grounds to get out so give yourself a nice long bath with bath salts. If you like, before you get out of the tub take a brief shower to help wash away all those released toxins.

DO YOU FEEL FAMISHED?

In all likelihood today's "rush to breakfast" is not about hunger. With all of the juices and broth you consumed throughout the day yesterday, your body has been fully nourished. Take a moment to think about your relationship with food.

Do you use food as a way of rewarding yourself?

Do you use food as a way of filling time and avoiding a real sense of purpose?

Do you use food as an excuse?

Do you use food for emotional soothing?

Do you use food as anger, sex, friendship, or entertainment?

It will make a difference in your life if you can acknowledge and name all the emotional undercurrents that drive your "hunger." Ask yourself, whenever you feel hungry, what it is you are hungry for, and see if it doesn't change your perspective.

THE DAY 2 MORNING MEDITATION AND BREATH WORK

You are beginning another day of the fast, and this meditation will help you reach out for some extra spiritual support—however you express your belief in a higher power.

Sit in a comfortable sitting position, back straight. Get into your meditational posture. Putting a little cushion underneath your bottom always helps. Lean slightly forward and rest your arms on your knees, palms open and facing upward, index finger and thumb touching each other so very gently to keep the energy circulating. Follow your deep easy breaths—inhale, stomach out, exhale, stomach in—and just allow yourself to really let go.

> *See yourself walking down a beach with me.* Just take a peaceful long walk, picking shells, seeing the beautiful sights of the shore: the myriad colors of blue in the sky, the blue-green gray of the ocean, the caramel tan of the sand. With every step into that giving sand, feel a sense of renewal. Feel hopeful. Feel how the rhythms of the earth and the waves recharge your battery. If you have loving memories of any physical place, bring those feelings along with you as you walk. Yes, it's safe to bring them here.
>
> *Down the beach, in the distance, you can see a large, beautiful ship at the dock.* As you approach the dock, you see a mound of exotic, ornately woven, and handpainted baskets of all kinds. You need to choose one, but choosing is not entirely easy because what you see in front of you are some of the most exquisite empty vessels you have ever encountered. Take your time, and pick a basket that best represents your inner beauty and style.

Holding your basket with one hand, hold my hand with the other and come aboard the boat with me. On board this ship there is all that you will ever need. Let us begin in the room of abundant wealth and security. Here, there is gold, silver, gems, cash, stocks, and bonds—more than you could ever use in a lifetime. Fill your basket with as much of this wealth as you need right now, knowing that the ship and this room will always be there for you to revisit and replenish your resources.

Walk with me to the next room. You will discover emotional abundance, a place where you get nurtured, soothed, and satisfied. Here you are unconditionally accepted. Take as much as you need. Nothing is heavy, and the space inside your basket is boundless.

The third room is full of spiritual reverence. Standing here, you feel at peace, accepting of your world and of your life. You are grounded in purpose, complete. Fill your basket with many gemlike perfume bottles filled with this sense of awe, tranquillity, and mystery.

Move on into the room of creativity. This room is overflowing with artwork, music, literature, instruments, equipment, paints, pastels, and clay—all kinds of artistic endeavors and materials. You can feel your own creativity resonating within you in this room. Let yourself be that artist you have always been, yet never fully explored. Collect the canisters of brilliance you need to express that artistic genius inside of you. Fill up with the cans of courage you will need to soar as a creative spirit. Revel in the beauty of inspiration and fill your basket full.

Come with me into the next room, the room of loving relationships. See yourself in an intimate loving relationship and be comfortable in that arrangement. You are exposed and vulnerable in your intimacy; this encourages the free flow of who you and your partner really are to each other. This kind of relationship is the most beautiful expression of human emotions. See yourself sharing laughter and passion, dreams and aspirations with this person. Express your fears and find that your lover comforts and supports you, holds you and caresses you. Dance the dance of a whole relationship in this room. Breathe it in. Imprint it all in your heart, soul, and mind. Take a photograph, or film it to take with you. Create an audiotape so you can hear it as well as see it. Promise yourself that you owe it to yourself to live it.

Come now into the room of accomplishment. Observe your life's experiences projected before you on a screen. You have found your purpose here on earth, and now see yourself fulfilling that purpose. Watch yourself enjoying your life's journey, enduring pain, encountering obstacles, struggling and conquering them! See yourself act with courage and grace. Come into the center of your whole being and know that you have come here to do a job and that you are doing it well. Make a tape of the film you have just seen. Make an audiocassette, a CD-ROM, and a video. Put them all in your basket. They must come with you.

Finally, the last room you visit on the boat is the room of grace and faith. This is a space that gives you the understanding that your life has meaning and timing; everything that happens reflects this fact, whether or not you can always comprehend it. See a desk in the middle of the room and a piece of paper on that desk. Go to the desk and pick up that piece of paper. On it is the answer you will need when you are most in trouble. The paper will be blank until you really need that answer. But when you do really need it, the answer will be there to serve you. Put it in your pocket and know that you have it and that it will keep you safe. As you leave this room, know that the people in your life were meant to be there, and the experiences you have were meant to be. This is all so you can fulfill your purpose. You can reach your epiphany, touch your own chords, sing your big song, dance your dance, create your painting, and, most of all, move in balance and in keeping with your own inner timing.

Depart the ship with your full basket, feeling complete in every possible way. Be confident that you can return at any time. The ship will always be there for you, the rooms will always be there for you, and there will always be abundance within each room for you. Coming back along the beach now, you experience this place in a very different light. Notice the difference in your heart. As you feel fulfilled, your desire to serve and express your true generosity has deepened as well. Notice how this beach is a complete act of nature, whether the day is blessed with a brilliant sun or a fearsome hurricane. This beach exudes the grace and honesty of nature. Destruction alternates with restoration, but nothing ever takes it away.

We are like this act of nature. No matter how much we strip away, damage, or mishandle ourselves, we revive and rebalance until we reach an even keel. Even if we leave ourselves behind, we can go back and be restored with a beautiful grace.

On your second day of fasting, *come out of your meditation with recovered faith.* Imprint your body with this knowledge and let it give you a beautiful poise.

Take deep, easy breaths. Connect with all parts of yourself from your feet to your toes to your knees. Feel the tingle as you make these contacts. Feel the breath move by your belly, abdomen, and heart. It clears the back of your throat, going behind your eyes. Let your vision be cleansed and peeled away like the skin of an onion, revealing deeper significances. Let whatever thoughts that come just gather around you. Feel buoyant in the peaceful and contained stillness.

THE MORNING DRINK

PINEAPPLE-PAPAYA-STRAWBERRY (pages 237–38)

Your morning drink is the same as yesterday, but the experience doesn't need to be the same. Let yourself get lost in the colors and textures of the many fruits. Watch the blender as these ingredients get whipped into one gorgeous melody. Set the table lovingly, with a fresh flower in your vase. Put on gentle music, or open a window to hear nature's music. Then sit down and relax.

WORKING WITH YOUR JOURNAL

Get your journal out and take it with you into your sacred space. Today is the day where one door closes, but the next one hasn't quite opened. Faith is the bridge to carry you through this day. Faith in what you are doing; faith in the higher place that has brought you to this day. And your journal is one of the most important keys to finding and holding that faith.

Begin by turning to a fresh blank page and writing the word "FAITH" in large capital letters at the top of the page. Underline it. Now write it again, this time even larger. Next, write down today's affirmation: *I surrender to the bigger picture.* Pause for a moment, and think about what you have just written.

Write about everything in your life that increases your faith. Write about the faith you felt as a child or the faith you feel as an adult. Where do you go to find and replenish your faith? Where is the place in you where faith lives?

Right now faith is what you are using to construct your vision of the future. How does your future feel at this moment? If you feel your vision of the future shifting, write that down. Right now, you are constructing the bridge you will walk across in your dreams tonight, reaching the other side by the time you open your eyes tomorrow morning. You need to move toward that place of trust if you can, knowing you are really a master bridge-builder.

MORNING WALK

Be sure to take a fresh bottle of water with you to keep you hydrated. Take in the morning air and push out the stale air with strong, confident breaths. Take in the environment. It is different today than it was yesterday. Identify as many changes as you can. Noticing these changes connects you to the cycles of life, and encourages the cleansing cycle you are experiencing within your body.

THE MID-MORNING DRINK

Choices:

Pineapple-Pear-Lemon (recipe page 240)
Grape (recipe page 239)

As you sit down with your Mid-Morning Drink, feel the *chi* strong in your body from today's morning work. Close your eyes and try to identify each of the distinct flavors that have been combined in your drink. Then visualize them holding hands to become one stunning beverage.

MID-MORNING BREATH WORK AND YOGA

This morning, choose a breathing exercise that suits the way you feel.

- Connecting Breath—cleanses you (page 120)
- Alternate Nostril Breathing—balances you (page 130)
- Fire Breathing—releases surging emotions, anxieties, and agressions (pages 165–66)
- Push Breathing—pushes more toxic material out of your mind and body (page 140)
- Angel Breath—gives you a jolt of energy and exhiliration (page 164)

Give yourself five to ten minutes of breath work before moving on.

Yoga—Day 2

Just the word "yoga" should bring you comfort today. Think about the word, and return to that refreshing space, that sphere where you are protected in a white circle of light.

Today as you do your yoga (see pages 221–36), be as loose in yourself as you can. Don't worry about perfecting form. Just do the poses and let them release you. Today's exercises restructure the body and the mind in a gentle, giving way. I call them my nonviolent demolition crew, because they break down the old and clear the way for the construction of a glimmering new edifice that will be you.

TODAY'S LUNCH DRINK

CARROT-CABBAGE-APPLE (page 241)

Juicing is a beautiful meditation. The process is alive and full of color. As you prepare your lunch drink, don't stand outside the process as a detached observer. Really throw yourself into it (the process that is, not the juicer). Imagine yourself absorbing the different colors through your fingertips—there is nothing more beautiful than the rainbow of colors you have in front of you right now. Take the time to smell every piece of produce before you put it in your juicer. Each piece has its own distinct fragrance, stunning and inspiring. When you drink what you've prepared, you know that something gorgeous and live is being created inside of you.

TEMPERATURE TAKING

I take my emotional and spiritual temperature on a regular basis. I ask myself how I'm feeling. I check my breath to see what it's doing. Does it feel tight and constricted? Right now, you are at the midpoint of your fast. How do you feel? Are you nervous about what is still ahead. Sometimes the only way to help yourself through difficult times is by living them one small step at a time. One hour at a time, one activity at a time, one prayer at a time, one breath at a time. I always tell people to take it *one juice at a time.*

AFTERNOON ACTIVITIES

I like to divide this part of the afternoon of Day 2 into two segments.

Segment One

Do something restful and centering. You can nap or just lie down. You can do a guided meditation of your own invention (or repeat one of mine) either in silence or with soft background music. Consider taking a bath with an essential oil. Neroli or vetiver might be nice. And, of course, there is your full menu of breath work to choose from.

The key is to not exert yourself, but rather to allow the juices you have infused into yourself a chance to do their work. Practice your Rooting Ritual (pages 235–36) if your anxieties become too much, or purge some of your anxieties with vocalization exercises and screaming.

If you get restless this afternoon, address your agitation by answering it with softness. Don't put up a wall or show a clenched fist. Try responding in a way that is gentler than you would normally, and see what happens. Whatever activity you choose right now, put the thought in your head that you are committed to the detox process. Even if you're feeling shaky, consciously connect to the idea of it, and try to put it out there in whatever you do. The thought doesn't have to have the strength of an oak tree right now. Let it be an acorn and know that is enough.

Segment Two

The second part of your afternoon is going to focus on getting the lymph system moving. If you're near a beach or park, get out of the house and head in that direction, doing some brisk walking. If you're at work this afternoon, find some stairs to climb or an uncongested sidewalk to strut your stuff. Take a bottle of water with you, adding a squeeze of fresh lemon. If you're fearful, or wrestling with headaches, take the water plus a combination of green apple juice and sea salt to sip on (see page 244). With the lymph system energized, you'll be picking up the pace of detoxification. While you're outdoors, try to find a large tree. Stand next to it and realize just how much this tree has endured. Take a little of that strength for yourself, connecting to nature and accepting the energy it can give you.

TIME FOR YOUR JOURNAL AND YOUR JUICE

GREEN VEGETABLE DRINK (pages 239–40)

I often take my journal out while I'm drinking juice. This may be a good afternoon for you to learn this habit. When you take out your journal, don't reread your earlier material, just get writing again. Try the following exercise.

Making Peace with the Past

Everything happens for a reason. Now is the time to confront and accept those reasons so you can let go and move forward with fewer burdens.

Use your journal to consider memories from your past that are troubling you—*at this very moment*. Opportunities you feel you missed. Losses that still haunt you. Decisions you regret. Don't go searching. Just write down the ones that are on your mind today. Keep your language concise. Now, next to each item on your list, write down a positive opportunity, experience, or development that was created as a direct result of it.

Let's say, for example, that the issue gnawing at you is your divorce. You know what you lost, but what did you *gain* from this experience? Did you gain self-esteem? Internal strength? New friends? A more loving relationship? A beautiful dog? Write your answer down and look at it. Understand that you are who you are today *because* of the difficult challenges in your life, not in spite of them. Let the necessity of each of these experiences give you faith that everything really does happen for a reason, and that even the darkest moments give way to growth, expansiveness, and a more fulfilling life.

Before you close your journal, look at your list and accept responsibility for the places you've been. Then let it go. The act of letting go and releasing your feelings about the past can keep you from making similar mistakes in the future.

CONNECTING TO THE *E* WORD

This afternoon I would like to recommend your first enema to remove toxic accumulations that may be backing up and weighing you down. Don't make a big deal out of it. Just follow the instructions on page 89 and let yourself be amazed by the relief this simple process provides.

DOING NOTHING, AND DOING IT WELL

It took me a long time to learn to sit still and do nothing, but I did it, and I'm proud of it. And if you get nothing else out of this program, I hope you too will have mastered this skill. Try sitting on a beach and staring out over the ocean, or sitting on a park bench looking at a tree, or just sitting on the living room couch or a chair. Guilt-free nonactivity.

ANGEL BREATH

Before dinner this evening, try the following breathing exercise:

> First, stand up straight. Keeping your arms close to your body, fold both arms, take both palms and press them up against the bottom of your chin. Inhale deeply while raising your arms, moving your elbows away from your body, as though you were spreading your wings. Your head will go way back. Pause momentarily in this position. Now, slowly, exhale completely, bringing your "wings" down into the body and dropping your chin to your chest. Feel the strength this brings.

After ten Angel Breaths, continue connecting to your energy source by activating the body along the energy meridians. Take one hand and gently slap yourself up and down the sides of your legs, from your ankles to your groin, and then up and down the insides of each leg. Slap the back of your neck, and then travel lightly down your spine as far as you can reach. Now go up and down your arms, inside and out. Really concentrate on bringing the circulation back into your body. Rub the soles of your feet firmly with your palms. Now rub your palms together until you can feel them warm. Close your eyes and place your warm palms over your eyes. Let the warmth clear up your vision and clear away any unwanted images. Next, take your hands and massage your scalp vigorously to wake up the brain with blood and oxygen and warmth. Then try massaging your outer ears until they feel slightly warm to the touch. Finally, finish this exercise by bringing your warmed hands back to the heart.

A PREDINNER THANKS

Sometimes before I have my evening broth, I pat my body all over with a lightly damp cloth. This wipes down the pores, opening them up fully to receive the change in air from day to night. As I tingle all over, I realize the existence of my body all around my emotional and spiritual core. As these feelings surround you today, remember to thank your body for working with you so well and being your absolute best companion.

THE EVENING MEAL

WARM VEGETABLE BROTH (pages 241–42)

On Day 1, I encouraged you to make enough broth for all three fasting days. As the evening arrives, you may be very glad you took out that insurance policy yesterday, preferring sleep or meditation to any evening kitchen work on Day 2. You have earned a very special evening. It is a remarkable thing to be so close to the end of Day 2. So serve your broth, and make each sip a celebration of this achievement.

A JUST DESSERT

Cap off this long day with one of the dessert recipes on pages 242–43. On warm summer nights I often put my Dessert Drink in a thermos and take it to the beach or to a park. What feels like the most comfortable place for you to be this evening? Under the stars? Under the security blanket of your own roof? Under the sheets, surrounded by pillows? Pick your spot and relax with your special beverage choice.

FIRE BREATHING

Before taking your bath tonight, imagine yourself as a dragon, powerful and fired-up. Think of yourself being charged by the heat and energy of the sun. As you hold these images in your mind, I want you to move through a series of short, powerful exhalations, pushing out through your nostrils with your mouth remaining closed. Start slowly, but try to pick up speed, moving toward short, fast, powerful exhalations, one after the other in rapid-fire succession. You can do as many as twenty-five. During these breaths, you will be inhaling passively through your nose but paying almost no attention to this part of the breathing. If you need a place to focus, focus on your stomach muscles. They are toning and strengthening as they work to push the air out. Sometimes I'll press my right nostril closed with my right thumb and Fire-Breathe through only one nostril. Then I'll hold my left nostril closed with my left thumb and Fire-Breathe through my right nostril. You could call this Alternate Nostril Fire Breathing. I don't call it anything, but I know that it gives me not only a strong clearing but also a boost of energy.

EVENING COMFORTS

Tonight, in your bath, bring out everything you have: candles, incense, bath salts, scented oils, bubble bath, sailboats, and rubber ducky. Release yourself into the water, and invite health, change, and faith into your body, your psyche, and your spirit.

Much of the detox and healing you have done today will be completing itself as you sleep tonight. You want to support this in every possible way, and that means coddling yourself. Lavender and chamomile are calming essences, so maybe you will add them in with the salts or oils. If you are looking for extra energy, rosemary, basil, and peppermint will give you a zingy shine. And if you have a touch of the blues, essence of grapefruit, tangerine, or bergamot might help. Use the bath as a beautiful temple whose purpose is to answer only your needs.

Tonight you might want to play some music in your bath, or sing a song of your own making. Create a meditation. What do you need to hear from yourself that would calm you down, move your energy, inspire you, or instruct you? Let these words be your meditation. Maybe you need a spoken word piece. Who would you talk to right now for strength and faith? Role-play a little. Imagine yourself to be this or that person, past or present, personally known or not known. But always come back to being you.

You might think, "This is so unlike me to do this" or "What if someone hears?" Do everything you can to insure your privacy, then pick these concerns up off your chest and put them to the side. This is your playtime, your cleansing fun camp, your arts and crafts, your show and tell. Enjoy this chance for complete and delightful inhibition.

When you are finished with your bath, stand in front of a mirror and ask yourself: "How did I do today?" This is your time to admire and praise yourself for today's effort and achievement.

A Healing Meditation Exercise

After your bath, lie flat on your bed and do some deep easy breaths. Move into a rhythm of inhale, stomach out, exhale, stomach in. Put your palms on your stomach and feel the pattern. Now squeeze your feet tight, all toes together, as though you were squeezing a lemon. Put all your energy into your feet. Squeeze them tight, tighter, tightest, until you get to the source of your energy. Then release, and let the energy flow out. Get into your calves now, and flex those calf muscles. Squeeze the muscles of your calves as tight as you can until they are the exact center of your energy. Release again. Move into the kneecaps and squeeze all the energy into your knees. Source it into the caps as liquid. Hold it. Hold it. Hold it one second longer, then release your energy and feel it flow out.

Travel now to the center of your belly, and fill up this place with your energy. Tighten the muscles, make them firm. Then hold that energy, knowing it is your source. Hold it and hold it and hold it, pleased with your strength and vitality. Create the most beautiful washboard. Then make it fluid again, and release the energy.

Bring your energy up to your heart now, bathing your beautiful, pink, beating heart with life force. Turn to this heart that has been so fragile in your lifetime and infuse it with vitality, giving it stamina, passion, and joy. Hold the energy there for a very long time, in a very strong way. Hold the intention of faith in your heart and open it up to a loving universe. Find your commitment to serve your heart well and hold it in this space. Ever so slowly, let the energy become fluid to move on.

Your throat chakra is next. Bring in that energy and strengthen your voice so that you can unleash it. Feel the energy give you the confidence to scream, cry, shout, or whisper whatever it is you want to say. Hold that intention in your throat for a long time, and feel the joy of opening up your voice.

Move your energy to your eyes now, going up behind them, all around them, and squeezing them tightly shut. Collect all of the pictures these eyes have seen—all that has brought you joy, brought you marvel, and brought you pain. Gather them all. And squeeze these many images into one drop of juice, one precious tear, a symbol of your past. Then open your eyes as wide as can be and let that tear drip out.

Finally, gently shift your focus deep inside your head into the brain. Gather all the thoughts you've ever had—and the thoughts you're having right this second—and gently squeeze them together. Squeeze them together till they become one ball of thought, then release this ball. Let it roll slowly down your body, across the floor, and away. And just feel your body as empty, yet still full, knowing the paradox of that balance that resides within you with such grace. Remember this grace as you exit slowly from this meditation to make your last preparations before sleep.

REMEMBER YOUR DREAMS

Ask yourself on this night to dream of beauty, courage, or strength. Or ask yourself to dream the answers to questions that still challenge you, and to remember those answers when you wake. Make sure to keep your journal by the bedside tonight in case you want to wake up and write during the night. It would be great to write just a little bit now—even if it's simply a wish of pleasant dreams—to mark the end of this essential day.

Give yourself a message to remember your dreams. If you have a dream stone, put it under your pillow.

And as you close your eyes for sleep, think of a special treat you can give to yourself after your third day of detoxification has ended. I don't mean food. I mean something truly special that could help you hold on to and develop the new you in a larger, more committed way. Maybe it could be a room in your home you will dedicate permanently to your process—your own little spiritual space, your own little temple. Maybe a leather-bound journal to document the next phase of your life. Maybe a small keyboard to accompany you, support your creativity, and encourage your new voice. Maybe a collection of new books to help you explore the edges of your experience.

Use your developing new self to think of something special, and promise it to yourself as a reward for your hard work. Then allow yourself to drift off to sleep, feeling truly extraordinary for your accomplishments. In spite of all the challenges, you have completed Day 2, and tomorrow you're going to Get Juiced! Sweet dreams to you now. You've done a magnificent job.

DAY 3 MENU

Hot Water and Lemon

MORNING DRINK	Pineapple-Papaya-Strawberry (pages 237–38)
MID-MORNING DRINK CHOICES	Pineapple-Orange-Strawberry Apple-Pear-Ginger (pages 240 and 238)
LUNCH	Cabbage-Carrot-Celery (page 239)
AFTERNOON SNACK DRINK	Green Vegetable Drink (pages 239–40)
EVENING MEAL	Warm Vegetable Broth (pages 241–42)
DESSERT DRINK	Berry Cobbler (pages 242–43)

Water and herbal teas can be enjoyed throughout the day.

12

Day 3: Getting Juiced!

It's the day you've been waiting for. If Day 1 was the day of changes and Day 2 was the day of challenges, then Day 3 must surely be the day of synthesis. From the very instant you move from dreams into consciousness this morning, you feel the difference in you. You're brimming with energy, strength, elation, and empowerment. Where you once experienced resistance, you are now experiencing eagerness. Where you once worried about fasting for a single afternoon, you may now be fantasizing about fasting for a fourth day. Talk about feeling different! Today you know you're going to make it through!

WHAT DOES IT MEAN TO FEEL FULLY ALIVE?

Today, you should have the answer. You are in your own skin. Connected, clear, and clean, you are alive in every fiber of your physical and spiritual being. One of the most impressive payoffs on Day 3 is the change in your strength and energy. You've laid the foundation so you can begin experiencing yourself as alert, present, and powerful. Today will prove to you that you have the ability to accomplish extraordinary tasks, and to make ordinary tasks extraordinary.

Something else you are going to notice, something new you are going to see the moment you look at yourself in the mirror this morning: your stomach is flatter than it has ever been. It's a modest side effect of the fasting process, but a dream come true for many of us. This, by the way, has not happened because of weight loss. It has happened because you have abstained from the kinds of foods and food combinations that make the stomach bloat: wheat, for example, sweets, and proteins mixed with carbohydrates. And, though your stomach is empty, you will not be feeling hungry. Another marvel.

THE FINISH LINE

You are approaching the end of your three-day journey, but don't get ahead of yourself, and don't rush the process. You need to stay calm, and to be with this day, to complete the full cycle of cleansing and healing. Stay with the fast and all of the supporting exercises and rituals, and attend to every detail with even greater focus than before. Day 3 will deliver a new you, but only if you are fully present.

Day 3 is a day of integration. On the first two days, you became acutely aware of your body's feelings, your mind's layers of complex thought, and your spirit's sense of higher purpose. Today, realizing that you are indeed going to complete your three-day fast, anxieties and fears melt away. In this new peacefulness, you will be able to fully experience the balance that exists within you, between the part of you that gives nurturing stillness and the part of you that is filled with vibrant energy. You are beginning to understand what it means to feel balanced and whole. On this day, you really connect to the process of "exchange" that started on Day 1. Exchanging the actions that brought you to this fast for the actions that will carry you forward into a more gratifying place, you are able to look back at your accomplishments and see forward to envision the future. Today you are a free person, owning your own words and your own actions. You express the "no" and "yes" as you feel it. You work with the big picture, letting heaven and earth blanket you in your actions. In this space of the third day you are freed from the bondage and responsibility of the past. You can create a future starting with the moments of the present, letting them build naturally, not in a rush, into a joyful existence as big as the sky.

You've done a lot of housecleaning on this fast, but cleansing is an ongoing process. Let the energy of your new and revitalized cells communicate in their own time to all of the cells throughout your body. Let them spread the message. The others will come along given time and support for your new way of being.

Your intention for today is to get juiced.

You've come into your energy in such a powerful way that you may not even *want* to break your fast tomorrow. You will, but part of you is ready to keep going, like the Energizer Bunny. Going and going and going. What's going on? It's simple. This is just one small sign that you are really getting juiced. The most joyful part of the ride has started. You feel decidedly in a deciding mode. A fix-it mode. A planning mind-set, ready to plan next week and next year. Many of the people I've worked with feel so strong and energized that they start making plans and intentions for what they want to do with their lives. Where did all this high-voltage energy spring from? You may have doubted me before, and you may have doubted yourself. But today you know. It isn't a dream and it isn't an accident. You have released so much old, made room for so much new, it is no wonder that you are truly juiced. And in this new, balanced energy state you will accomplish your dreams.

Today's affirmation:
"I am the energy that flows through me."

As you take in your affirmation for today, it enters you without a challenge. You know it is true, and you can feel it instantly penetrate your heart chakra.

Life feels seamless today. You are at a high point of integration, and there doesn't seem to be any separation between what you want to do and what you actually do. Today is one of those grace days when life doesn't get any better. Enjoy these feelings, but don't burn yourself out. It's a gift to feel energized, but it's also a gift to treasure that energy and not feel like you must do, do, do.

Our culture has been so programmed to be on the go that the moment we feel energy, most of us feel we have to *do* something with it. Understand that it is enough just to feel this power, and that you will use it in *your* own time and in *your* own way. Today simply exist where you are and be satisfied. The future is coming, and it will be wonderful, but happiness revolves around the present. Don't miss out on it. Sink into the synergy of this day, as mind, body, and spirit meet, greet, and join.

Don't disrupt this moment. The temptation is to bounce out of bed and bounce into activity, but that will not honor this day. Instead, remain in bed this morning for longer than you usually would—at least a full fifteen minutes longer.

Take notice in your body of what it feels like to have this movement of true energy. Feel the newness, feel the aliveness, but hold your center and remain calm.

BREATHING IN THE NEW DAY

Lying in bed this morning, place your palms on your stomach and begin deep easy breathing. Let all parts of you connect. You can almost see your heart extending a hand to your stomach, and both extending a hand to your brain. A perfect circle is completed, as the mind, body, and spirit hold hands within you.

I want you to try to breathe consciously all day long today so that inhaling and exhaling engage your entire body. No more shallow breaths that nourish only a fraction of your cells. Full and complete breathing will help you in all of your activities today and in the future.

Whatever you choose to do today, make a point to stay present and engaged, and try to extend the activity five or ten minutes beyond the point at which you would normally stop. Exercise longer. Meditate longer. Scream louder. Stretching like this lets you get a sense of your elasticity and growth. You have the energy, and you have nothing to be afraid of, so push your edges just for this day. You don't want to spend your life pushing yourself beyond your place of balance, but when things seem fixed, immutable, or locked down, your memory of this day will remind you that there is always room to expand.

Add a few deep breaths today when you are in bed. Find your center, your still point, and stay in it. This is the place from which you will take all further steps; the place from which you will identify all doorways that lead to the rooms you need.

THE MORNING RITUALS

- *Hot water and lemon*
- *Morning skin-brushing*
  Skin-brushing has become such a part of you that you may find yourself getting lost in the process, turning it into not only a cleansing, but a meditation.
- *Morning bath*
  As thc waters rise around you, swirling with bath salts, tub toys, and essential oils, drop further into your peacefulness. You don't have to be tranquil. Oh no. You can sing, you can splash, you can arrange your ducks into a bright flotilla, or you can wave your arms and pretend you're a tropical fish. Whatever you do, make this bath a time of celebration. Look and appreciate the body that you have. It is beautiful. It is praiseworthy. So go ahead and give yourself a compliment out loud. It doesn't matter what you say. If it's winter, when you're finished with you bath, you can add some organic sesame oil or olive oil to a damp washcloth and use it to moisturize your body.
- *Morning drink*
  Pineapple-Papaya-Strawberry (recipe pages 237–38)

DAY 3 MORNING MEDITATION

Get into your comfortable meditation position and begin this morning's meditation with a very deep breath. Use that breath to let out any of the anxiety that you've been holding the past two days. You may still be experiencing some of the physical symptoms of detox, such as itchiness, bad breath, flatulence, and the like, but they are already dissipating and you now know that they will pass.

Take deep easy breaths. 1–2–3–4–5. Recall the image of your body, mind, and soul holding hands, creating a circle in the center of your body.

> *Imagine now a pinwheel*—when you were a child you might have gotten one at the circus or at the five-and-dime. And when it caught the wind, all the wheels turned and the colors swirled. Bring that image back now. Pick a beautiful green pinwheel—greenish yellow—and imagine that swirl of color and energy spinning in your stomach. A gentle breath, and it swirls around the center of your stomach. Hypnotic.
>
> *Move now to your heart*. There I want you to see a pink pinwheel. Take another breath and gently blow to start that pinwheel turning. Watch it turn. Watch both turn, the green one and the pink one, like an amusement park within your body.
>
> *At the top of your head, the center of your forehead, the crown chakra, there is now a beautiful violet pinwheel.* Watch it pick up the wind of the other two pinwheels and start to spin. Watch all the wheels spin and let this vision stimulate you. It is your energy that is moving all of them. Watch these wheels spin into the center of your system, feel its vitality. Continue to nourish and detoxify with deep, even breaths. Let all things toxic that are moving out of your body continue on their pathway out, through your skin, through your hair, through your breath, through your thoughts. Just let them squeeze out of your body, through the air, through the pinwheels.
>
> *Through the connection of the pinwheels, bring wind, air, and light into your body*. Let this vision allow a spontaneous creation of spaciousness inside of you. Embrace this space, and give it permission to enter into your home, your relationships, your job, your whole outlook.

Let it give you a new set of eyes, thoughts, words, and actions. Feel inspired by this spontaneous openness to bring a spirit of creativity into everything you do.

DAY 3 MORNING WALK

Some people are so eager to get physical on Day 3 that they want to turn the Morning Walk into the Morning Sprint or the Morning Marathon. If you are absolutely driven to doing this, then okay, do it. But it is more important to try to channel your energy into noticing the world beneath your feet and all around you on this great day. And this is more successfully accomplished at a moderate pace.

WHERE AM I NOW?

This morning is a great time to sit down with your journal and free-associate about what you are feeling and thinking at this moment. Write down: "What action could I do for another person anonymously?" Use this morning's clarity and start writing down everything that comes to mind. Good feelings, intentions, plans. If you have kindness, compassion, and clarity inside you, the hardest work has already been done. Why not look into yourself now and experience the joyous discovery of all that is there?

THE MID-MORNING DRINK

Choices:

Pineapple-Orange-Strawberry (page 240)
Apple-Pear-Ginger (page 238)

TODAY'S YOGA

As you practice your yoga (pages 221–36), open your heart and feel the harmony in your body. All connections should be made through the heart. Let everything you are feeling filter through your heart and experience the internal connections this sacred art helps you complete.

THE LUNCH DRINK

CABBAGE-CARROT-CELERY (page 239)

I like to do everything I can to invite the spirits into my life on Day 3. I light some incense near the table, then close my eyes as I sip my lunch drink. As the waves of flavor roll over my tongue, the scent of the incense creates a soft, airy mist around me. It's dreamy and inspiring.

Stay with this special moment, merged with all of nature's vitality and brilliance. Your intention for today is to get juiced, and here you are right now, literally, emotionally and spiritually doing just that.

TODAY'S AFTERNOON ACTIVITIES AND YOUR "CHOICE LIST"

Your choices:

- Silent time
- Nap time
- Do nothing
- Enema (at some point today, you should definitely take your second and final enema) (page 89)
- Screaming it all away (pages 94–96)
- Walking meditation (page 93)

LETTING GO RITUAL

Go into your sacred space, get comfortable, take a deep connecting breath, and imagine yourself taking a walk with me through your house.

> *It's time now to take a walk to the place in your life where things are stored*. Imagine a basement where many boxes can be held. There are so many boxes here, and you need to look at them now, seeing them all piled up in front of you.
>
> *In one very large cluster of boxes are papers filled with all of the promises made to you in life*. Promises made to

you by parents, teachers, lovers, friends, and bosses. Promises made by magazines, newspapers, movies, television. Promises made by new situations—new jobs, new relationships, new homes. Promises of all the things you were going to have, going to be, going to do. They are all in front of you now. And you want to start opening those boxes and reading those promises.

Read the promises. And let yourself experientially go through what you were told, what you believed, what is in you, what you still hope for, what you pray for, what has disappointed you. Hold them in silence while you read them. Let yourself have these promises. Retrace them once again. Take all the time you need.

In another area of this basement is a second cluster of boxes. And in these boxes are papers filled with all of the promises *you* have made. Promises you made as a child who believes in a joyful future. Promises made to schools and to parents, to brothers and sisters, your first boyfriend or girlfriend, your partner in life. Promises made to your job, your career, your talents. Promises made to charities and to people on the street. Promises you've made in passing. Promises you've made on vacations, resolutions, New Year's Eves. All the promises you've told yourself, about yourself, to accomplish this day, this month, this year, this life.

Read through these promises now. See where you have met yourself and where you have not come to meet yourself. See where you have been disappointed in life, let down, dismayed. And see where you have surpassed yourself, experienced things you could have never imagined, attained achievements far greater than you could have hoped for. Revel in the accomplishment. Bring together the promises you made with the promises that were made to you. See where they meet, where they are the same, where they have become one voice.

When you have integrated all voices—your many voices, and the many voices of others who spoke to you—it is time to close up the boxes and start stacking them. There is a door that leads outside. You see a crack of light. Open that door, see the light streaming in, and start to carry your boxes outside through that door. Pile your boxes in a tall circle. Now *imagine* taking a roll of newspaper into the center of this circle and lighting it on fire. Use this imaginary torch to light all of your boxes in the circle. In your imagination, burn all of your boxes in a dazzling circle of light and heat, and watch as the flames consume this part of what was your life. Watch it all burn, all the thoughts you held energetically, real or imagined, from people or from yourself. *Bless this flame as it is burning because it has made you what you are at this moment.* Now it is about to synthesize and transform you into another part of yourself. It is giving you a new muscle, a new thread to follow into a better life. And after the fire has burned down, see the clean space that has been created in the ashes. You are free of promises now. Clear of past obligation to anybody and to yourself. You are free and clear to start over completely new.

And with this sense of liberation, return now to the beautiful pinwheels you know are inside of you. Look at the pinwheels, calm and beautiful, and know that you can activate them at any time with your breath and your silence. Return to the pink pinwheel that is your heart, and see it pulsing and open. Receiving, vulnerable, and soft. Come back to the yellow-green pinwheel in your stomach, into that place where you have the power to generate your energy.

In these three pinwheels that are yours and yours alone, you have your complete self: clean, forceful, moving to the pulse of your own breath's beat, your own personal tune. And now, having connected again with these three parts of yourself that are always within you and reaching for each other, take three easy, complete breaths and ease out of your meditation. Breathing in, stomach out; breathing out, stomach in. Wonderful.

From this moment on, you have passed through the gateway to your freedom—freedom from all the selves that have owned you before.

BREAK FOR A SNACK DRINK

GREEN VEGETABLE DRINK (pages 239–40)

In the flurry of your afternoon activity, make sure you take a fifteen-minute break to enjoy your juice.

ESSENTIAL JOURNAL TIME

Choices program the mind to help you look for what you want. If you consciously make a choice, you program the memory of your choice into your being. So then when things happen in your life, a part of your memory will always be engaged to say, "Yes, this is what I choose," or "No way!"

As you return to your journal this afternoon the first thing I would like you to do is make a Choice List, a list of all of the things you choose to happen in your life from this day forward. Each item should begin with the words "I choose to. . . ." You might write things like this:

"I choose to live in joy and freedom."

"I choose to have abundance in my life always."

"I choose to turn my will over to powers greater than me."

"I choose to have a portion of my life devoted to service.

"I choose to be committed to my purpose in life."

"I choose good health."

"I choose to have a beach house and a red convertible."

"I choose healthy relationships."

"I choose to take three vacations a year."

All of these things are choices you have the power to make for your future, and you can make them right now. You are not reaching for the impossible here. This isn't about fantasy. You are choosing to put healthy possibility into your life, and stating to yourself and the world that you are willing to work with these goals.

Start with the Basics

If you are having trouble getting started, focus on very basic things first, such as food. As you have learned over these past three days, basic choices like foods ultimately make the larger, more complex choices possible. You might write, for example, "I choose to eat really well." Then get specific, listing all of the foods you want to spend more time with in your daily diet.

What about emotional attributes? What do you need to fulfill the many parts of yourself? Perhaps you might write, "I choose to be kinder, more patient, compassionate, and truthful in my life." Or "I need to understand and dismantle my anger so I can be more open to feeling love."

Start a fresh page in your journal when you are ready to explore the area of relationships. On Day 3, the balance you have found gives you a very profound insight into relationship issues. It gives you an inside track, and makes you feel more powerful in this very perplexing arena of life. If you are not currently in a relationship, use this time to explore the lessons of a recent relationship, or the lessons of being with yourself. If you are in a relationship, this is a good time to take stock and examine its significance.

AFTERNOON REST

Many people feel an energy drop at this time of the day because they have been doing so much emotional, spiritual, and physical work. Even if there's more you need to get done, don't try to push yourself through this point. Instead, lie down and let your body revive itself naturally.

MAKING THE TRANSITION INTO EVENING

Whenever I reach this point on the third day I always feel like the mountain climber who, after gargantuan effort, is finally in a position to see the view. It is both exhilarating and gratifying, and I use my breathing exercises to "inhale the view"—to center me on the huge picture that has unfolded in front of me and help me digest it without feeling overwhelmed.

Choose whatever breath work speaks to you most right now. Your choices are:

- Connecting Breath—cleanses (page 120)
- Alternate Nostril Breathing—balances (page 130)
- Fire Breathing—releases surging emotions, anxieties, and aggressions (pages 165–66)
- Push Breathing—pushes more toxic material out of your mind and body (pages 140–41)
- Angel Breath—gives you a jolt of energy and exhilaration (page 164)

After ten or fifteen minutes of breath work you might want to sit in absolute silence for another ten or fifteen minutes. Let the silence allow you to fully experience everything that surrounds you and that you feel in the deepest parts of you. Feel the joy and feel the peace. When you have finished, feel free to record in your journal any additional insights or feelings that have come to you as you make your transition into evening.

HAPPY HOUR

ORGANIC MARY COCKTAIL (page 241)

This is one of my favorite treats during a fast. I like to put this drink in a really festive glass with a stalk of celery. You have earned this delicious celebration, so enjoy it to the fullest! You can lick the celery, but don't eat it. Consider it your first flirtation with solid food.

DINNER IS SERVED

WARM VEGETABLE BROTH (pages 241–42)

Whether you're making a new broth again tonight, or warming the broth you prepared two days ago, I'd like you to add a sweet potato to the mix and let it cook in there for a while. I want you to add the sweetness because tonight is about sweetness. You are approaching the end of Day 3, and little touches like this reinforce the sweet feeling and help make it memorable. Wear something extra extra special to dinner tonight—something you would wear out for dinner on New Year's Eve, or out for dinner in a tropical paradise. Light candles and take the time to appreciate how stunning you must look illuminated by the gentle flickering of those candles. Let your evening and your mood stretch out.

EVENING DESSERT DRINK

BERRY COBBLER (pages 242–43)

If you can handle a dessert drink tonight, do it. Try to go outside into the beautiful evening air with your drink, even if you have to bundle up tight. Toast the world. Look up at the sky and search for stars. No more giant-screen TVs for you. Today you have found the bigger picture, and you have mastered a process that will always bring you back to it.

EVENING COMFORTS

Tonight you want to take a very long bath, warm, soothing, and sacred. Light candles and incense—sandalwood, frankincense, myrrh, or patchouli would be best. Transport yourself with exotic music. Take yourself away with the new energy of you. The sounds of nature, whether they are trickling in through a small crack in a window or surrounding you courtesy of a CD player and a great nature soundtrack, are going to help you connect to the many spirits of the natural world and their energies. All kinds of spiritual connections are made and strengthened on Day 3. Moving through a portal into a more spiritual realm has given you a taste of a new world, but it is for such a short time. You may be concerned you are going to lose the thread, and that it is going to slip away all too fast.

The best way to meet these issues is with stillness, balance, and calm. So sink into your bath now and ask the water to penetrate your cells with its liquid purification and float away the remaining toxins. Sink, release, and be still.

Imagine you are on a really fabulous journey with your new self, feeling lean, taut, and tight in your body. It's a journey to the forest . . . a playground of adventure for your soul. Invoke the spirits of your animal self, the animal energy that speaks to you most. Maybe it's a butterfly for transformation, a dove for peace, or a bear for strength. Let these spirits travel with you. When I go on this journey, I always imagine shamans coming to greet me and take me through. There is a male and a female, to give me balance, and I imagine they are coming to take me through the forest to initiate me, to bring me through a special rite of passage into some portion of myself that I have not met. Try to imagine that you too have these mystical guides, and that they will take you to meet the part of you that is fearless, fully energized, crystal clear, and most sacred.

As you travel, you can sense the meaning of life in its entirety. Plants and animals all feel so close to you, and you can see how everything in nature works together so well. It's a natural circle of communion and you get to watch and be a part of it. Frogs and flowers, water and wind . . . you watch them work together. Colors, sounds, textures, energies, all working together. You are now part of that composition. It makes you feel truly blessed: special, but also humble, recognizing that you are just one small part of this rich fabric.

Surrender yourself to this oneness. Let yourself feel accepted, trusting, and safe in this inspired community. You do not have to feel isolated anymore. You do not have to feel separate. Replenish your cells with oxygen, breathing in and out with the many plants and animals. Let the green that surrounds you fill you with its life force. Relax in the lushness of nature. You have entered the forest, like every other animal. Have no regrets, guilt, or doubts about who you are and how much you will always be connected to this way of life.

At the end of this bath, spray yourself with a cool shower to tingle, stimulate, and awaken your body. Dry yourself with real vigor. Put on wonderful oils. I especially love verbena, patchouli, tangerine, and lavender.

PREPARING FOR BED

Your mind, body, and spirit may all be very busy in your dream life tonight. You are processing your accomplishments and preparing for your future, but it is also very important that you sleep well, rest, and rejuvenate. To assist you tonight, you may enjoy placing some crystals under your pillow to energize the healing process. I use hematite for dreaming, and I also use rose quartz to open my heart.

Keep your journal close to your bedside tonight, and be sure to have your pen handy as well. Tonight, you may wake up more than once with exciting new thoughts filling your head. Instead of letting them steal your sleep, you can jot them down quickly in your journal to release their spell on you and return to them in the morning.

Some people will be feeling so exhilarated late into the evening that they cannot imagine sleeping tonight. But you do need to sleep. So, if you are one of these people, make yourself some calming herbal tea. Practice some of your most stress-releasing breath work. Try to write your way into a less charged state, using your journal to help purge and contain any conflicts, questions, or excitements. And consider using a meditation of your own design to bring you into closer alignment with sleep.

GOING SOFTLY INTO THE NIGHT

When you are ready for bed, lie on your back and put a hand on your belly and a hand on your heart. Take five easy, deep breaths. Picture the hands connected again—heart, stomach, and brain; soul, body, and mind, and feel the union. Part of you is already preparing for tomorrow, the first day of the break-fast. Soon, you will release into the changes this day will bring, but right now, you need to acknowledge the beautiful feat you have just accomplished. Three days of doing everything new. A new way of eating. A new way of feeling. A new way of seeing. A new way of being.

Thank yourself for seeing you through this magnificent cleansing journey. Now thank each part of you for its contribution. The parts of your body all showed up, listened, learned, and did the hard job of rejuvenation. Now you know how to empower yourself, from the deepest place. You know how to take yourself through the most stressful times, and through immense change, and do so in such brilliant form.

So give every part of yourself thanks tonight, and acknowledge the participation with a series of gentle pats. Make little pats everywhere on your body, pats of congratulation for a job well done. Start by patting your forehead, at the third eye. Move to the nose, the eyes, the brow, the cheeks, the mouth, and the chin. Gently pat your throat, your chest, and the region above your heart. Move to the stomach, the intestines, and the groin. Move down through the thighs, the knees, the calves, the ankles, and down to the bottom of your feet. Gentle pats for every part of you. A job well done.

Acknowledge the sweetness in you, and prepare for the sweetest of dreams. You have witnessed the miracle of life. Three days in labor, and a new human being has emerged. Tonight you are a newborn once again, shiny, shimmering, fresh, and alive. Soon you will walk back into the world as a different person, meeting others in a whole new way, and leaving behind so much of what you have needed to shed. This is the stuff that the sweetest dreams are made of.

13

Breaking the Fast

JOURNEY PLUS ONE DAY

Today you are at a critical juncture. You have cleansed your body, mind, and spirit to a polished shine. But the cleansing isn't over. It will continue to go on depending on how much detoxing space you allow yourself today, tomorrow, and for the rest of your life. You have outfitted yourself with a whole new set of skills for tuning into yourself, others, and the world around you. Use the time, energy, and love you have invested in yourself these past few days to mark not an ending, but a new beginning. You are free to be a new you.

Breaking a fast is the most important part of the entire fasting ritual, and the first few days of that break-fast are crucial for the body you have healed, for the psyche you have liberated, and for the spirit you have celebrated. You need to go forward with your life without sacrificing your newfound personal power and integrity.

PROTECTING THE NEW SPACE YOU'VE CREATED

When you started this process, I told you that because of the cleansing process you were going to create new space. And you have. Now what we want to do is make sure that you use that new space to your advantage. Giving your break-fast short shrift can undo many of your hard-won gains. I'm not just talking about running off to satisfy your first food craving. You can undermine yourself in much subtler ways. I'm talking about every aspect of your life that has been cleaned, cleared, and sorted. You need to approach the world gently, because right now, too much too soon of anything will send you into a spin.

This chapter will help you understand how you can hold on to what you have learned these past few days as you make the transition into your day-to-day life, and how you can build from there. It all starts with an attitude, and that attitude begins with the word r-e-s-p-e-c-t. Respect this breaking the fast transition period, and acknowledge it as a significant link in the bridge to the new you.

WAKE UP AND SMELL THE NEWNESS

For the past three days, you were fully engaged in a very structured program. You were always busy—even if being busy meant sitting totally still and clearing your mind. It's going to be different today. Of course I have specific food suggestions—that's very important. I hope you continue with your hot water and lemon, skin-brushing, bathing, and daily breathing exercises; they are all wonderful things that I would like to see you integrate into your daily life. The most important part of today is that it's a day of Free Choice. There are no requirements—only modest suggestions. You gave me three days to lead you, but today you are back in charge, and the only structure from this day forward is a structure that is going to come from you. The future is yours, and it's a future you have been waiting for a very long time. I sincerely hope there will be rituals and attitudes that you will incorporate into your life. Take what you want and need from the program; it's up to you to decide what that is.

This program is about progress, not perfection. The structure you need is within you now. Your cells have been imprinted with a new plan for living. Stay centered and balanced and remember the wisdom of this journey.

WHAT CAN YOU EAT? WHEN CAN YOU EAT IT?

Let's start by focusing on the first day of breaking the fast. Your body is still getting the message of healing. It's in a new mode. And you may not be hungry, at least not for the foods you've always craved. You have to come back gradually into the way you eat. Your eating habits may never be quite the same again.

As you realize how certain foods like dairy, corn, or wheat affect your body, your clarity, and your moods, you may not want to eat them anymore. Or you will eat them fully conscious of the consequences taking place as they rattle through your system, and find ways to minimize their impact. You may, for example, eat less of the things you once loved. Or you may eat them at different times of the day than you did before, because you know your body is stronger at these times. I am hoping you will drink a lot more juice and a lot more water. I am hoping you will buy organic foods whenever possible. Frankly, I am hoping that you will "do food" differently in all kinds of ways, but we'll leave that to the next chapter. Right now, we need to talk about breakfast.

IT'S TIME TO START CHEWING

The best way to break your fast is not to feel guilty about eating. Believe it or not, you may feel as though there is a betrayal going on. This is normal, You may feel suddenly let down when you start eating. Your body is starting to transit. Start this day with the Morning Drink. You know how to do it, and it will help prepare your system for what's next. You may be pressed for time today, but try to take time out to relish your drink and hold a spirited connection to the past three days.

About an hour after your Morning Drink, it's time to begin *slowly* eating *small* quantities of solid foods—high-water-content fruits, to be specific. So start. Cut up some fresh organic papaya, watermelon, and/or pineapple, or take a cluster of seedless grapes. Chew slowly and carefully. This is the wake-up call to your enzymes, which have been resting for three days. Really delight in the chewing as you taste the new flavor. Your body has been resting, and you don't want to shock it with big solid pieces of food. You want to give the enzymes in your saliva lots of time to do their predigestive chores.

Thorough chewing is an excellent practice, always. You will be amazed at how much your digestion, nutrient absorption, and elimination habits improve from just this simple act. You will also be amazed by how much pleasure you can get from every single bite of food. You'll appreciate it more, enjoy it more, and need much less to feel full and satisfied. If you feel a little bit guilty about going back to solid food, remember the balance part of the fast. Food is a necessary part of life.

If you know that you won't have time to make your Morning Drink today, you can make it the night before and freeze it. Then you can take it to work, take it to school, take it to the airport—wherever you have to go—and let it thaw naturally along the way.

WATER BREAKS

You need to drink a lot of water today, and you need to be drinking it throughout the day. Don't return to the tap. Drink mineral water—six cups would be great, eight cups would be even better. People who are returning to work tell me it's hard to drink this much water on the job, but then they'll down cup after cup of coffee or drown themselves in diet sodas. If you can't get good water at the office, take some from home. Add a squeeze of lemon or lime to perk things up.

A GREEN LUNCH

For lunch today, eat a green salad. Don't yawn, be inventive. Get as many different kinds of organic produce as you can find: arugula, romaine, chicory, mâche, chard, watercress, dandelion greens, etc. Speak with your local produce person to help find the freshest and most flavorful stuff. Chop your greens up into bite-size pieces, toss them all together and then squeeze some fresh lemon on top to dress it. As you assemble your salad, imagine that you have a job at The Gap, decorating a spring window, filled with shades of green. Take small mouthfuls and chew slowly.

Help your body remember what it feels like to have solid foods.

For lunch, you also want to have a big glass of fresh vegetable juice. Carrot juice is probably the simplest to make, but you have all kinds of choices from your newly found juice repertoire. Ideally, you want to prepare your juice just before you drink it. If you will be at the office today, or won't have the time at midday, make your juice in the morning (or even the night before, if necessary). Unlike the fruit juices, vegetable juices lose their "life" if they are frozen, but you can refrigerate your juice if necessary, or put it in a thermos to keep it fresh.

EVENING MEAL

For dinner, prepare a wonderful bowl of steamed organic vegetables. I love including zucchini, string beans, broccoli, cabbage, cauliflower, carrots, and a little bit of sweet potato. Make your own choices; just don't overload on the squashes. You can sprinkle your steamed vegetables with seaweed flakes, tamari, or even Bragg's Liquid Aminos. If you like, add some fresh ginger.

If you're in the mood for an appetizer, cook up some more of the Warm Vegetable Broth (you might even have a little left over from yesterday). If you prefer, you can turn the Warm Vegetable Broth recipe into a hearty dinner. Then you've got an evening chunky vegetable soup that brings back fond memories of your fasting days but also gives you something good to chew on. If there is any leftover broth, freeze it and use it later to cook your grains.

After dinner, you might want to relax with a cup of tea. Spearmint and licorice are two of my favorites during the breakfast. And now you can add a small spoon of honey, or even a little bit of date sugar. But don't use any regular sugar right now, not even brown sugar. Your body isn't ready for the jolt. Tea is not your only option tonight. If you liked the carrot/celery nightcap you had during the fast, you can juice up some more tonight and let it calm your nerves. And of course, hot water and lemon is always an option. I try to end my evening with hot water and lemon regardless of what else I choose to drink.

WHAT ELSE WILL YOU DO TODAY?

You may need to return to these worlds you left behind, but you don't need to return at your old pace, or in your old way. Whether you are a corporate CEO or a full-time mother of five, one of the biggest challenges of today is bringing as much of what you have learned during the past three days into your first day back on the job. It starts with what you eat and how you eat it, but it doesn't need to end there. Brush your skin. Take a relaxing bath (if you can't do it in the morning, do it at night). Practice your breath work whenever the opportunity presents itself. Consider taking a yoga break after lunch. And try to go *slow* today. Not just when you eat, but with everything you do. Drive slower, walk slower, talk slower. I know this is not an easy thing. Things move pretty quickly "out there." Sometimes the only way to meet this fast-paced world is to hold your own slow, steady pace. You know the benefits now, and your behavior can be an inspiring example to others.

This is a good day to put yourself in a "witness" mode. Notice everything you are doing. Try to stay in the moment and watch or witness how you talk, how you behave, how you think. This is always a good way to maintain a spiritual frame of mind.

TAKE SOMETHING NEW TO YOUR ALTAR

Spend some time in your sacred space, and reflect on new ways of being and doing that you can take to your altar. New ways of being with yourself and new ways of being with others.

If you like, you can add something concrete to your altar to symbolize integration back into your daily world. It doesn't have to be elaborate. Just meaningful.

SET ASIDE TIME TO MEDITATE

I said before that I have no structured program, other than the food program, to offer you on this day. I do have one other thing to offer you, though: a last meditation to bless and reinforce your reentry process. Think of it as a graduation present from me, and please try to find twenty minutes in the morning or afternoon of this day to present yourself with this gift.

If you are at home, use your sacred space for this meditation. If you are at work, take a break and try to find a space that is quiet and feels private. Sit outside if you feel like it. Sit in your car if that's comfortable. Use your office if you can turn the phones off and keep people from knocking. Do what will work best for you.

THE BALLROOM MEDITATION

Sit down and get comfortable. Sit cross-legged if possible, resting your arms on your knees, thumb and fingers touching. Deep, easy breaths bring you into what your being is feeling like—clean, healthy, energized.

> *Move with me now into a giant ballroom with large mirrors all around*. The room is glittering and shiny, and you're so excited to go inside. As you walk into this ballroom, pause in front of the first mirror, the mirror closest to you. This is your physical mirror. Take time now to look at yourself, viewing the body you have, not the body you want to have, or you should have had, or you had before. Really look now at your real body and be with yourself. Experience each curve, each muscle, each inch of substance, and allow yourself to love your body. Love and accept your body.
>
> *In the next mirror, let yourself experience the ideal body you think you want*. Step into the future and create. See how your legs would be, the height, the tautness of them. See your abs as tight as you want them. A washboard stomach if that's what you want. Do you want to have curves? Or do you want to have long, sleek lines? You have a picture in your mind. Everyone does. You've had it for a long time. Now is the time to conjure up that picture.
>
> *In this same mirror, see how the inside needs to be in order to reflect this outside body*. What would it take within

you to make this body yours? What kind of attitude? What kind of discipline? What kind of lifestyle? What kind of eating habits? Instinctively connect with that interior self. If it makes you happy to be there, commit to making a bridge to move into that new interior and exterior self. Be willing to change some of your habits. Make a mental, emotional, and spiritual picture of this interior/exterior self so that every day, on the unconscious and subconscious level, you are journeying toward making that picture real in you. Be peaceful about this. Don't make it an enormous pressure or effort. Just be focused and consistent.

In the next mirror you see yourself in a world context. Observe yourself working and creating, doing everything you have wanted and always said you would do. You are completely accomplished and at ease. Visualize who you are meeting, what you are meeting about and where it is all happening. Absorb the satisfaction this experience brings to you. And if you don't know yet, if it hasn't come to you in life yet, open yourself to this information right now. To do this, first relax and let your mind clear. Then let it go to a place of purpose. Instead of asking the question, "What am I going to do in my life?" allow your life to come into you. As you stay open enough to allow life to come to you, watch the picture as it fills in. Become that picture. Release the notion that a goal is all-important, that it is both the end and the means. It is really just one part of your life's rich soup. See it in its place, in balance. Stay with this mirror, in this mirror, until you have absorbed this information into yourself.

Move on to the next mirror, the mirror of satisfying relationships. See yourself in perfect harmony with another. Let new relationship waters open up for you. Take hands with this person who meets you here at this point of departure, this point of new beginnings. Look into this person's eyes. Embrace. See your emotions connect. Think of the people you trust the most now. Put them into this person, knowing that the trust and the love fit together as you both do. See how you feel safe in this profound touch. Build your relationship future from this moment. Leave your history behind.

Turn next to the mirror of your spirituality. Find where you turn to when you have used up all your own resources, when you are frightened, when you are doubting. This may be an energy, or your God, or your goddess, or your animal spirit, or all of nature. Deepen your faith in this mirror. Acknowledge how this essence protects and surrounds you on a daily basis. Know that it has a destiny for you to be joyous, happy, and free. Know that it is there, even if it cannot be touched or seen, only felt. Connect with and surrender to this power and your destiny with it. Relax. Allow your hands to let go of all that you are grasping to control your life. Free-fall into this encompassing, glorious protection.

As you walk to the end of the ballroom now, you smell wonderful fragrances. There is a room filled with roses, peonies, and lilacs, and a myriad of other flowers of every color and scent. Sit in this room and let your senses come alive. Open to your hearing and hear that people are speaking to you. Open to the power of your voice, knowing that you can be strong and centered, even while being soft and gentle. Open up your eyes and see beyond what people are saying and doing to connect with what is right in front of you. Then see even beyond that to the most precious point in life, to what is really important. Gather all of this sight and let it become a part of your vision. Now go with this into the third eye in the middle of your forehead. Open up your intuitive channels. Open up your real knowing, the part of you that always knew, yet didn't follow. Open it up and ask it to join you on your new path. Tell it that you'll be able to follow it easily now. There is no wrong action to take anymore. Everything you do will be right.

Stay now in the third eye in the middle of your forehead. Experience how the universe is all there. Feel the expansiveness within it. Open the top of your head to the bluest and biggest sky and let your head be filled. If clouds pass by, just witness them. Let the sunshine balance your brain, the fluids of your spinal column, and reverberate in you. Take the flowers in the room around you and toss them high into the air. Have the petals float down and adorn your entire body. Reexperience the joy and play of your sensual self. And when you feel vibrant and vital, slowly start to come out of the meditation and back into your body.

There is a happy, tingling sensation now at the bottom of your feet and throughout your body. Fill your belly with new enzymes, energy, and integrity that you haven't had in your system in a very long time. Sense how your organs have a synergy with one another. Move up into your heart, purring like a satisfied kitten. Slide into your throat, up to your eyes, your nose, your ears. Feel the energy and aliveness. Allow your thoughts be still. All is well. All will be well.

FOOD SUGGESTIONS FOR THE SECOND DAY

The second day of your break-fast is another important day. Your system is starting to readjust to solid foods, but you are still in transition, with one foot in both worlds. Fight any cravings that may be surfacing as you leave your home today, Believe it or not, the typical food craving, no matter how intense it may feel when it hits, usually passes in less than thirty seconds. Breathe through your cravings. Only thirty seconds of willpower and that stranglehold, that "I can't live without this" feeling, slips away. Don't take my word for it—take out your stopwatch and see for yourself!

THROUGHOUT THE DAY, BE CONSCIOUS OF WHAT YOU EAT

Breakfast

Start the second day of your break-fast with another filling glass of that old reliable Morning Drink. If your elimination system is still sluggish from the fasting shut-down, this would also be a good morning to have six or eight organic prunes (let them plump in water for thirty minutes before you eat them). But don't eat them just because I said it's okay. Make a conscious decision as to whether or not it feels as if your system could use the assistance. From now on, you want to consider *everything* you put into your body, whether it's good for you or not-so-good, full of fat or fat-free, totally organic or coated with resins. You don't want to eat *anything* on automatic pilot anymore, even if it is something as fabulous as your Morning Drink. This is part of what it means to become food-conscious, body-conscious, and life-conscious. For several days, I have made all of the decisions for you. It's time for you to start making those decisions.

Once again, feel free this morning to chew on some high-water-content fruits such as grapes, melon, or pineapple. Take your time and stay focused on each bite. You want to establish a new relationship with all foods, and it begins each morning with the choices you make to start your day. Try to appreciate the life and "personality" of everything you eat.

Lunch

Lunch on the second day of your break-fast should be a baked potato or yam (no butter or sour cream yet, please), and a green salad. You can also have a baked squash—butternut or acorn. Add a few slices of avocado, tomato, cooked beets, or broccoli to your salad if you wish. If you have saved some broth or vegetable soup from last night, and would prefer to have that for lunch, that's fine too. Just try not to load yourself up. You want to feel filled, but not stuffed. Filled means taken care of; it means satisfied. Stuffed means over the top. After you chew each bite of food or sip each spoonful of soup, assess whether you really need to have the next one. With each mouthful, you are checking to see how much you need to replenish your cells and retain balance. Your body will give you all the information you need to make these decisions if you keep that channel open and assure your body that you will respect this information.

Dinner

If your energy level seems good and you're still feeling clean, start introducing some protein back into your system. Some people will be primed for protein earlier, and they know they will be able to handle a little bit for lunch. That's fine, as long as you don't have protein at lunch *and* dinner. Personally speaking, I prefer to wait until the end of the second day, but everyone is different and the choice is yours. Just try hard to let this choice come from within your body, not from staring at someone else's hamburger at work today.

For today, not every protein is okay. Keep to tofu, tempeh, or fish. And if you're having fish, steer clear of fatty fishes like salmon—the fat content is way too high for you to handle right now. Think more in terms of sole, halibut, or flounder, and try to stick to what is fresh, not frozen. It would be terrific if you could find fish that had been caught the same day you are buying it, so check around at your local farmer's market or fish market if you have the time. Cook it simply, without sauces or butter. Grate some ginger, add some tamari, and bake it at 350 degrees until done—about thirty minutes. Whatever you choose, keep your portions very small, take small bites, and chew each bit thoroughly.

If you don't feel that your system is ready for protein yet, don't force yourself to have any today. You don't *have* to start eating protein yet. So trust the internal signals, and finish your day with steamed vegetables and rice, or steamed vegetables with some other grain. If you want to have rice, use basmati rice. Brown rice is just too rough when you are coming back into eating solid foods. If you want a different grain, don't use anything processed. Go for the pesticide-free choices and consider trying something a little different like quinoa, millet, or kasha. These are all lovely cooked up in your leftover vegetable broth. You can also brown some onions and add them to the cooked grains for a wonderful added flavor (they are also excellent for assisting the digestive process).

Continue to keep corn and wheat out of your meals today. Both of these foods are not well-tolerated by many people, but the primary allergic reaction—sluggishness—goes unrecognized by people who are accustomed to feeling sluggish and unclear. Soon you can start experimenting with corn and wheat and see what, if anything, they do to your system, but today I want to keep you as clear and clean as possible.

If you want dessert tonight, have some fruit or some natural, sugar-free applesauce. In fact, you should try to stick to fruit all week. You *could* add whatever you wish, but I think you will find that when you are truly functioning in balance, you will actually crave fruit as a dessert and be turned off by the world of desserts you left behind.

Activate Your Digestion

One last thing. Twice today—one hour before lunch and one hour before dinner—it would be great if you could take two tablespoons of apple cider vinegar (mixed into a glass of distilled water). This will get the peristaltic action in your gastrointestinal system going and help reboot your digestion in a very natural way. Taking apple cider vinegar twice daily will make a marked difference for you in your ability to continue detoxing after the fast. Ideally, you should continue this practice for two full weeks after the fast. Many people make it a permanent part of their daily diets.

RITUAL, EXERCISE, AND MEDITATION ON THE SECOND DAY

Is there anything else from the fast that you can carry with you into this day? Hot water and lemon in the morning? Journal-writing in the afternoon? A soothing bath at night? What about some yoga, some breath work, or a brisk walk? Do what you can to create a spiritual bridge from your fasting days into your daily life.

If going to your sacred space has helped clear the path for you during the three days of fasting, consider making this contact a part of your daily ritual. Use it as a place to meditate or write or rest or make a dedication. Every day I make a dedication at my altar. If there is something specific I'm trying to accomplish I will write it out and put that piece of paper on the altar. I keep some beautiful handmade papers and an antique fountain pen at the altar to use exclusively for this wish-writing. And the simple act of returning to my altar every day continues to change my life.

EATING SUGGESTIONS FOR THE REST OF THIS WEEK

On the third day of your break-fast I still recommend starting with fresh fruits and/or a Morning Drink. Green salads are best in the afternoon, and veggies and protein for dinner. On the third day, you can start bringing in chicken, turkey, lean beef (organic if possible) if you want it, and fattier fishes like salmon. On the third day of your break-fast, and for the rest of this week, the important thing is to try to keep your meals simple and "clean." Clean means not too many foods at once, as opposed to five-course banquets that run the range of your refrigerator's contents. Fruits and juices in the morning. One meal of lovely vegetable salads. The other with steamed veggies and protein. If you can eat your larger meal at lunch, it would be wonderful. For example, protein and salad at lunch; grains and veggies at night. Keep your choices limited and clean.

Clean also means small portions. You're better off eating four or five small meals than loading up for winter each time you sit down at the table. Smaller meals keep the burden off your digestive system and keep you feeling light and clear. They help you gauge your true hunger, they increase your awareness to your positive and negative food reactions, and they also keep you from falling quickly back into old automatic eating habits that might not be healthy, or even satisfying.

It's as if you have been on vacation and you're coming back to your house. You can't do ten or twelve things the moment you return, even if they are all there to be done. You look at the mail, but you don't open every piece. You check your answering machine, but you don't return every call. You do a little. You rest. You do a little more. You rest. You take out the garbage. You phone a neighbor. You feed the cats. But you keep it as simple as possible, addressing only one or two things at a time. Sooner or later, everything gets taken care of without sending yourself into a spin.

As you leave your liquid vacation and walk back into solid food, you're going through the same kind of scenario. The key to success is small, simple meals. If you are easily overwhelmed by food and need a place to focus, focus on protein and vegetables for the rest of the week. You especially need the protein right now, even though you don't want it in excess. If you can handle it, try the "mono" eating approach (see page 113–14) to some of your meals. To remind you, mono eating means eating only one category of food at a given meal. For example: just fruit for breakfast, just vegetables for lunch. It may sound strange but it can really work to support your system by keeping digestion simple and focused. The more foods you try to eat at once, the more your digestive system has to "multitask." It can do it, but it takes a lot more internal energy and effort. Mono eating is like a low-level fast. You will probably find that you lose weight doing this.

Try to follow these suggestions for the remainder of the week, and, if at all possible, through the second week of your break-fast. You may be saying, where's my comfort food? Where is my pasta and bread? If life and work make it too hard to stick to these guidelines for more than a few days, just make sure your carbohydrate intake is minimal for the next two weeks, and your fat intake is even less. By now, you should be starting to think of carbohydrates differently anyway.

"LET THE SUN SHINE IN"

Plan something special for yourself one week from your first day of reentry to celebrate your success. Something other than food. While foods and fasting have brought you to this place, your achievement has brought you a different perspective on living that includes, but is so much bigger than, food. Let your celebration reflect the breadth of your growth.

Perhaps you could spend a day at the beach, in the mountains, or at a spa. Maybe you could give yourself an afternoon of massage, sauna, and play. You could shower yourself with gifts—

special music, beautiful craftwork, or lovely fragrances. You could enroll in a spiritual workshop, or you could go to Disneyland and stay there until the park closes! Whatever you decide to do, this is a day to be particularly kind and good to yourself. You have done what only you could do: allowed yourself to be you.

TAKE SOMETHING FROM YOUR ALTAR, AND TAKE IT TO ANOTHER ALTAR

In the last few days you may have placed an object or amulet of some kind on your altar. This would be a good time to take that object and place it on another altar. You can take it to a church or a temple. You might want to take it to nature and place it near a tree. Think of this as a simple act of energy transformation and exchange.

BODY HALF EMPTY, BODY HALF FULL

By fasting and cleansing, you have created a unique opportunity for unending growth. In a profound way, you have taken everything out of your system, achieving a kind of ground zero from which you can go forward in a very different way, learning about the continuing needs of your body, psyche, and spirit. This is the ideal time to take a moment to fully understand what you have done for yourself. The way you are now is your baseline. Because you are in balance now, you can see the way the rest of your life effects this baseline. From the food you eat to the people you know, ask yourself what helps you maintain balance, and what tilts your scales. Starting with food relationships, it is time to explore the nature of your interactions on every level, in every situation imaginable. From eating pasta, to doing sit-ups, to sitting in silence, to balancing your checkbook, to driving to visit your grandmother. Since you are coming out of a clean zone, you are going to see, more than ever before, what works for you and what doesn't. You can learn more about yourself in the few days and weeks following the fast than you have learned for years. All it takes is a willingness to trust your own experience. For the last three days you have paid your dues. Now all you need to do is pay attention. Check your reactions to wheat or sugar; notice what happens when you eat something that contains additives or preservatives. How do you know if something does not agree with your system? Here are some of the signs: feeling loss of energy, headachy, cramped, itchy, agitated, uneasy, angry, or spaced-out. Here are some more: feeling super-speeded up in a racing, unstable way, or diving into a bad mood. And I'm not just talking about food allergies here, I'm talking about "life allergies"—negative reactions to people, places, and things that just aren't good for your system.

The positive signs are just as important. Be on the lookout for things that make you feel strengthened, calm, light, happy, peaceful, centered, buoyant, or even energized. This is the "food" that your soul craves, and today the signs will be clear and obvious.

CHRONICLING THE NEW

I encourage you to record in your journal your reentry experiences from the first day of your break-fast forward. Your future is a flexible thing, a process of trial and error, experimentation and learning, challenge and growth. Understanding the impact things have on your well-being is a very powerful tool for your own growth and self-preservation. It better prepares you for difficulties, and it gives you clear positive goals to strive for as your life journey continues. Goals such as these: more time with your loving relatives and less time with others who are unsupportive; a job that involves fewer administrative duties and more fieldwork; more warm proteins and fewer chilled foods; more natural springwater everyday and fewer sweetened beverages; less direct sunlight and more filtered light; more time talking with your child and less time going shopping with your friends. You get the idea.

If you are paying close attention, you can learn about not only the obvious things, but also the most subtle, down to the smallest detail. By attending this carefully you might discover, for example, that every time a butterfly crosses your path you feel a little bit happier for days. Does this mean you should rush out and spend more time looking for butterflies? Maybe. Or maybe it will help you remember that, even though you don't have everything you desire, you can still find much reason in this world for joy.

Start experimenting, and make what you learn work for you. This knowledge is your richest inheritance, and it all comes from you. All it takes is careful attending. You can call it being centered, conscious, or being present in the moment. I like to think of it as being "on the observe." Life is about learning, and being on the observe means always being open to learning, and to the growth that learning brings. This is not to suggest that you are supposed to be just an observer of life, and not a participant. You should still feel totally free to do whatever you choose, as long as it is what *you* want for *you*. If you want to dance on the table, do it, but not because people expect you to be the life of the party. If you want to talk on the phone for hours, do it, but not because hanging up sooner might hurt someone's feelings. Do things for you. Let it reflect a concerted commitment of your mind, body, and spirit harmonizing together every day, every moment focused on your well-being. When you start to live in and appreciate each moment you have on this earth, you will be amazed not only by how much more you enjoy life, but also by how much more you accomplish and contribute.

14

Going Home Without Getting Lost

How will you meet your future? How will you integrate everything that you have learned and experienced on your three-day journey into your real life in the real world?

I know people who go to Europe and experience the time of their lives. They lose themselves and become different people. They eat exciting foods, they eat at different hours, they talk with interesting strangers, and sometimes they even begin romances with these interesting strangers. The real romance they are having is with the new people they have become. While they are on these trips, each person thinks the same thing, "This is the real me. How I wish I could always feel this way." Then, they come home, and suddenly a switch gets thrown. They shut down all of their openness, receptivity, and experimentation, and within days of returning home, they go back to being and feeling exactly the way they were before they left.

Right now you are probably very concerned that the same switch is going to get thrown inside of you. If you are afraid that the demands of the outside world are going to pressure you to abandon all that you have accomplished, you need to know right now that the choice is entirely yours. Entirely.

The fast may be over, but the real work has just begun. This is not a time to be giving up, it is a time to be gearing up. You have learned an important truth about yourself: You can go farther than you think you can. As we reach out for renewal, we realize that we are sensual beings who don't have to go through life anesthetized. In this process of rejuvenation, what you brought forth is a new sense of you and your future. You don't know what you will become; that's the mystery and wonder of the future.

THE BIG FOOD PICTURE

Because of all your diligence during the fast and break-fast, your cells now have a memory of what it is like to be free and clean. Yet there is still an emotional memory and attachment to food—and the wrestling match is about to begin. Part of you will crave health, while part of you craves ice cream. Part of you wants beautiful fruits, part of you still wants M&M's.

Relationships, holidays, stress, and rich desserts will shift your balance. But you've already touched your core so you have a center to come back to. This is the memory of a clean body.

So much of what we are surrounded by in Western culture focuses on perfection. From here on try to think about things differently. Try to become *choice*-oriented rather than goal-oriented. When you are really living life, you are always arriving. It is process that should never end and never be tiring.

FOOD FACTS FOR THE COMING MILLENNIUM

For the second week of your break-fast, you should to reorganize your whole approach to foods. What do you eat? For starters, make sure you are consuming a lot of protein. Many of us have spent the last ten years hypnotized by carbs. This is a new era, and it's time to build up the body, and watch the pendulum swing from pasta to protein. Protein is the new "buzz" food; it will make you lean, it will make you strong, and it will stop your cravings. It would be great if you could get your body back in protein balance. Two egg whites every morning would be excellent (once in a while, you can eat the yolk too); you could even try having miso soup and a small piece of fish or poultry in the morning and see how your energy level responds. Most of you won't be used to this kind of breakfast, but it's a great way to make you alert and prevent cravings.

For your afternoon meal have a piece of fish (minimize fatty fishes—see page 199), chicken, or meat. And at night you can have some selected carbohydrates—yam, baked potato—but even then I recommend adding some tofu, tempeh, fish, chicken, or meat. If carbohydrates have lost their magical appeal and you would rather have soup and/or veggies for dinner, that's great, but still have some protein too.

Protein is going to build your muscles, and you will burn off what you don't need. Keep your protein intake interesting by giving yourself many alternatives. If you are a vegetarian, pay close attention to your protein intake. Tempeh, rice and beans, and all kinds of tofu will do a good job for you. When you cook your beans, try adding kombu, a natural mineral seaweed. Cooking kombu in beans, as well as in soups, broths, and gravies is a great way to mineralize the body.

You should also consider using nori flakes, which are a good source of seaweed—and an excellent balance for UVH rays. Sprinkle them on everything—your rice, your soups, your veggie-burgers. Whether you're on the phone all day, at the computer, or running around town, you'll have the cleaning and fortifying power of seaweed working its magic. Seaweed is also excellent for your thyroid.

EVERYTHING OLD IS NEW AGAIN

With your reentry process underway, it is important to remember the many things from the days of fasting and early days of break-fasting that can help you every day from here forward. The *simplicity* of your eating habits during those days is one of the most important virtues to carry with you. But don't confuse simple with plain. Simple means that the food you eat is easy to digest. That means staying away from the kind of food that may look artistic on the plate, but is impossible to digest. Think about some of the complicated combinations that some restaurants serve.

Instead, opt for a simple one-plate meal by grilling trout seasoned with a squirt of lemon, tamari, and ginger, and complementing that with a big bowl of fresh garden greens dressed with olive oil, fresh lemon, cumin, and some fresh garlic. Try to stay away from yeast-producing dressings with mustard and gourmet vinegars. Don't deprive yourself, the meal should be a rich experience. I'm not big on deprivation. Eating should be an exultation of the wonderful flavors and textures and smells of food. It just takes a little creativity and courage.

Now that you're familiar with the juicing process, take a look at the range of juice remedies for simple ailments like everyday aches and pains. Some of them are so delicious you may just want to make them periodically for the taste, and to use generally as tonics.

In the second week of your break-fast, continue to try new things and try old things in a different way. Your Morning Drink is always an ally; maybe you'd rather have it for lunch now. Your broth maintains balance, keeping your system from being too acidic. You could bring some to the office in a thermos.

A CORNUCOPIA OF EATING APPROACHES

With your fasting and break-fasting complete, how will you approach food in the months and years to come? It's exciting that there is such a broad range of nutritional roads on which you can walk. Here are some of the long-term programs and systems that worked for me and helped me maintain balance as well as a comfortable weight. If any one, or more, appeals to you I encourage you to read more about it. Then adapt your choice and make it your own in a way that makes the most sense for you.

When you are traveling or in restaurants, don't be afraid to ask for what you want. Experiment, be flexible, be creative, go slowly, go wisely, go intuitively, and trust the healthier voices that have sprouted inside you.

Conversation about food appears to be the new sex talk of the decade. Everywhere I go it seems people want to talk about what they are or aren't eating. In my case, I really believe it helps me if I change my eating pattern a little bit on a regular basis. Every ninety days I add some foods, and stop eating others. I do the same things with the various supplements I take.

Whatever approach to food you choose, certain guidelines should always be the same: buy and eat organic wherever possible; shop frequently so that your foods are always fresh; eat slowly and chew thoroughly. You always want to remain conscious of what you are eating, and how it affects your always-changing rhythms and sensitivities. With these simple guidelines, you can be assured of daily meals full of energy and flavor.

Create a food chart to help you document your reactions to certain foods. It will keep you in tune with your system and its many reactions, and the help can be immeasurable. You will really begin to see how some things are good for you at one time of the year but perhaps not at another. You will see how your emotions and the state of your spirit affects your eating patterns and needs, and vice versa. You will see how eating foods that are not in season and have been warehoused or preserved can wreak havoc. This kind of writing doesn't need to be exhaustive. One or two words will speak volumes to you about what you can and cannot handle, what you do and do not need.

No matter what approach—or combination of approaches—to eating you decide are right for you at any given time, remember always to be kind to yourself; be flexible, be open, and even be comfortable indulging your cravings in moderation, understanding that they are a part of you, not a failing in you. This last point is particularly important. If your life and your eating patterns are balanced, then having a monstrous plate of barbecued ribs one night for dinner is not a federal offense calling for self-imposed exile. I've never been healthier since I incorporated the whole spectrum of eating—a little bit of dairy, a little bit of tea, a little bit of sugar. All of it.

I also need to say that it is your body you are living in. What goes in can stay in for a really long time—sometimes forever. So be mindful every day of what you put into your body or expose your body to. Always try to at least pause before you indulge in something that seems way over the top. Sometimes a simple pause is all you need to change your mind and make a healthier decision.

It's time to look at some of the healthful approaches to eating for your future. As you read through these approaches, remember that eating is an ongoing balancing act. You always have a choice. Exercise it.

EATING NATURALLY

Whole-foods eating helps us take advantage of nature's bounty as it was originally intended. It is a simple, natural path to healthy eating that automatically removes many of the toxic additives we have become too comfortable with in our foods. To engage in whole-foods eating you want to prepare and consume your foods in their original form. What would you eat if you were living on an island in the Caribbean? Whole-foods eating means staying away from foods that are processed, preserved, coated, or treated (which, of course, means *buy organic*). It means staying away from prepared, prepackaged, ingredient-heavy items. It means avoiding meats that have been raised with antibiotics and hormones.

The human body knows how to use whole foods efficiently, to supply nutritional, spiritual, and physical balance. The whole-foods approach is really quite simple: it encourages you to enjoy unadulterated, healthy foods, and enjoy them in a way that feels most congruent with nature.

FOOD COMBINING

From the standpoint of digestion, not all foods are compatible with each other. This doesn't mean that some foods are good and some are bad. It just means that not all foods get along together inside your body, and that this conflict can compromise your digestion and your health. When you organize and eat your foods in groups that are digestively compatible, you are doing what nutritionists call "food combining." The advocates of food combining say that eating foods in correct combinations will vastly improve digestion.

The key to food combining is arranging your daily diet so that the proper enzymes needed for digestion of a particular food can work without interference from other foods and other enzymes. If digestion is better, the system is cleaner. The cleaner the system, the more energy the body can obtain and expend. Following are some basic principles on food combining:

- Protein may be eaten only alone or with certain vegetables. Veggies can be any color or shape; they can be cooked or raw.
- Starches can only be eaten alone, or in combination with vegetables (cooked or raw). A little oil can be added for enhanced flavor.
- If you are eating dairy products, do not eat them with anything else. This means no milk and cookies; no yogurt and granola.
- Fruits and vegetables should not be eaten at the same meal.
- Always eat fruit at least one hour *before* eating anything else.
- Melon does not mix with any other fruits. Eat it alone.
- Do not combine more than two types of food at the same meal. Fox example, if you are eating fish and vegetables, do not eat bread.
- All beef should be eaten with an abundance of green vegetables.
- Do not eat anything sweet immediately after eating protein.

The above suggestions are meant to give you an idea of what the practice entails. There is a wealth of detailed information on food combining to be found in health-food stores, bookstores, and libraries. Check it out if you are the least bit curious.

SYSTEMATIC UNDEREATING AND FOOD CURFEWS

When you intentionally eat smaller portions and/or eat less frequently, you allow the body to activate and accelerate its natural cleansing functions. Systematic undereating allows for a clearing of stagnation in the digestive and elimination processes, which is a frequent cause of illness in the body. A really clean approach to eating in this fashion would be starting the day with miso soup with tofu, carrots, and scallions. Have a little protein at lunch and bring your carbohydrates in for dinner to get the relaxing effect they bring to the body.

It also really helps to finish your eating by early evening. I use 7:30 as my cutoff, and I actually try to eat earlier. This makes a huge difference in healthy digestion, regardless of *which* food approach you choose for your future.

You can systematically undereat as an overall food plan, three meals a day, or you can do a less comprehensive approach, such as undereating one meal daily. This could mean replacing one meal every day with a glass of juice, or with juice and a small salad. You could easily do this if you started each day with the Morning Drink, or if you had a Lunch Drink every afternoon instead of a big meal. Some people consider systematic undereating a rejuvenation approach that helps them maintain energy.

There is a glut of meal replacement powders on the market—from high protein to high carb. These powders are a great way to introduce undereating by a liquid meal replacement. Some people make them into smoothies or power shakes by adding herbal or nutritional support. There are also new beverages coming out called nutriceuticals, which are created by adding vitamins and nutrients to everything from juices to waters.

Do not try to systematically undereat if you view it as a weight-loss plan. This is not the purpose of this approach. Systematic undereating is a profound body-mind-spirit plan, not an "eat less and lose" diet. You might not lose a single ounce with this plan since your system will intelligently and intuitively maintain a balance within. A by-product of being clean and balanced is a body that is able to regulate its proper weight. Your proper size will find you naturally, and everything will be in its place.

THE FASTING TRACK

You have survived an extraordinary challenge: a three-day juice fast. For many of you, it was a first. Could you imagine a second? Or a third? Could you imagine an occasional one-day fast? A half-day fast? It's time to start thinking about the future, and thinking about fasting as a part of your future.

Periodic fasting keeps you connected to your body's natural tendency to cleanse and rejuvenate. The end of your three-day journey can also mark a vital beginning, a turning point in your life, a decision to commit to the fasting process periodically for ongoing healing and growth. Many people go on a three-day fast twice a year. Others fast at the change of each season. Still others fast one day or one half-day every week. What would work for you? All of these fasting regimes are powerful choices. According to some people, if you fast one day a week from sunrise to sundown, you might slow down your aging process significantly. If you could fast at the turn of each season, you would find yourself living a more integrated, balanced life that honors the cycles of the body and the cycles of nature. Try fasting once or twice a year, and watch it create a stability in your health, weight, and energy.

You have seized your own future. Let fasting help you make the most of it. As you think about your many options, keep the following pointers in mind.

Fasting Through the Seasons

The best times to do long fasts (three days or more) are the beginning of spring and the beginning of the fall. In the spring, the body is full of the salt and sugars it has held on to from the cold winter months. Your body has its own version of winter accumulation and you want to clean that out. You want to bring the green, growing life back into your body, and that makes your green drinks with parsley, spinach, wheat grass particularly valuable.

The fall is also one of the best times for long fasts. The body is getting ready to get quieter for the winter; slower breathing, less motion, quieter emotion. The Chinese say our ability to adapt to change is how we cope with disease. If you can cope with change, chances are you won't get sick. So you want to help ease the transitions. You want to help your body adapt and accommodate to the beginning of winter—and maybe even yearn for it as a time of rest.

It's fine to fast in the summer because there is such an incredible abundance of gorgeous fruits. If you're going to fast in the summer, make sure you stay well hydrated. I use lots of lemon and pineapple in my juices and dilute my drinks in the summer with water (50/50). Then I freeze them to take to the beach, to work, or wherever. As the drink melts, you get the sweet juices first, for the cleaning, followed by the water for replenishing. In the summer particularly, don't fast for more than three days. It's too much strain on the system.

Winter is the most complicated season for fasting. The calm bear in each of us wants to hibernate and connect to the earth, while our bodies are looking for extra insulation from the cold. If you choose to fast in winter, use lots of broths and herb teas. You can make broths from fresh greens, misos, and variations on the vegetable broth you made for the past few days. Potato-leek broth is great in winter, and my favorite is a root-vegetable broth with sweet potatoes, squashes, and beets. Experiment, and let your body tell you what it needs most.

YOUR BODY KNOWS WHEN FASTING IS BEST

People don't like to fast when they are experiencing a lot of stress, and the body doesn't like it either. After these stressful times have passed, however, fasting is the best way to recreate balance in your system. If your system is in upheaval, let it be in upheaval, even if that means more than one piece of chocolate cake with ice cream. But promise yourself that you are committed to bringing yourself back into health with fasting. Your body-mind-spirit will believe you, and it will take care of you.

Fasting is an excellent way to catch up, reorient, balance, and center after a lot of traveling. It is a particularly good antidote to airplane travel. Even a one- or two-day fast will get that toxic airplane air out of your body and reestablish your electrical system's proper functioning. When I know in advance that I'm going to be doing a lot of flying, I prepare a Morning Drink for the plane and try to stay as clean as possible. I don't get food phobic, but I do try to do whatever I can to keep my energy up and stay on track until I get home to cleanse and rebalance.

As you make fasting a more regular part of your life, you will notice that you are cleaning out more quickly each time. I have been fasting for seven years now and I can do a serious cleaning in just one day. In three or four days my system is absolutely pristine. There is no reason you can't feel the same way.

Remember that each fast accomplishes something a little different. Every time you engage in the process, the body establishes its own list of cleansing priorities, then tackles those priorities. Each time you will *feel* slightly different. More tired one time, more agitated the next. More filled with cravings one time, more filled with emotions the next. More severe one time, more mild the next. Always different, always changing, but always exactly what you need.

WHAT ELSE WILL YOU TAKE WITH YOU?

As you journey into the future, you now have fasting at your side. You also have other rituals: meditating, for example, writing, skin-brushing, bathing, and visiting your altar. And you have exercise: practcing yoga, for example, walking, vocalizing, and breathing. You have a new relationship with food. You have a new relationship with silence. You have a new relationship with nature. And you have a new relationship with yourself. You have enriched your life in so many ways in the past few days. Your task now is to keep it rich. To keep it filled with meaning, beauty, depth, and health. The choices are yours. And those choices will change over time as you change and grow. But your body has already learned everything. Your new cells carry the memory of your journey, and they will pass this on.

Don't overwhelm yourself with promises right now. Don't do that New Year's Eve thing that so many of us do, setting ourselves up for disappointment. The goal is to fill your future with life, but this is best accomplished with very small real-life steps. It takes a commitment, but only a commitment to keep trying.

Maybe you will start with some foods, maybe you will start with one or two exercises, or maybe you will start with a small ritual. Maybe you will spend an extra fifteen minutes each day making your breakfast more special. Maybe you will spend an extra fifteen minutes each day making your relationships more special. Or maybe you will spend an extra fifteen minutes each day honoring your creative talents. Maybe you will come to your altar every day the way I do.

The template for a new approach to your life is already in motion. The possibility has already opened doors and given your life a sense of expansion and possibility. Meet everything with the same openness that you feel now. Make this your intention for the future. The rest will unfold the way it was always meant to unfold. Perfectly.

Epilogue: The Truth, the Whole Truth, and Living in the Truth

At one time or another, all of us have felt sick and in need of some kind of healing treatment. The kind of treatment you receive depends very much on whom you approach to heal you. If, for example, you have chronic indigestion and go to an MD, he may say you have gastritis. If you go with the same symptoms to an Indian Ayurvedic spiritual healer, he or she may say that your *pitta* (fire) is too high, and you might be given some powders. A traditional Chinese healer may diagnose you in terms of obstructions to your "wind" and your *chi* (energy). Again, you might be put on some herbal regimen and perhaps some acupuncture. Energy healers from masseuses to shiatsu therapists to lymph drainage experts might attempt to access your energy by balancing the body with hands-on therapy. A new age MD might have anything in his or her bag from homeopathy to Prozac.

When I was at my sickest, I was like a broken-down automobile going from shop to shop until every mechanic in town had worked on me. Some were truly helpful; some didn't help at all. Some were confused; some were confusing. Some were kind; some were scary. Some tried their best and failed. Some were inspiring. Some were life-draining; some were lifesaving. Some "repairs" lasted years; others lasted minutes. Some found and focused on big problems; others found and focused on little things. And some stole my parts. These people taught me that a great deal of energy is being spilled on the sharp cutting edge of the healing movement. But there is also a lot of magic, a lot of hope, and even a handful of true miracles.

New Age spirituality is about an alternative approach to healing. The best part of this shamanistic approach occurs when the healer is able to encourage or invoke parts of your spirit to engage in the healing process. This can have almost miraculous results when the person who wants healing finds new energy which he or she is able to use as an empowering tool. Simply put, if you are seeing an MD for your gastritis, or your gynecological problems, and you have already invoked your own spirit to be part of the healing process, you're going to have better results than if you simply sit back and hand over your power. The important thing to remember is that finding your own healer or truth can help keep you well.

My life goal is to know the truth about who I am, however painful, uncomfortable, or fabulous that truth might be. I believe we all need to embrace everything we learn about ourselves at every stage, no matter what the outcome. For me, this is the only way to live a full life.

Living in the truth means being able to hear, see, feel, and honor the truth. Sometimes that's frightening, and it's always sobering because most of the time, living in the truth means change. Now I know that you are ready for change, and I know you are equipped to handle change. How do I know this? Because only people who are ready and equipped are drawn to this program. Our willingness to change is beautiful; it is the warrior in us all. And I applaud each and every one of you for thinking that maybe, just maybe, you could do this. *Maybe* is the biggest word in our vocabulary, the word that opens each new door. And through that opening, we enter into growth and a fuller life.

I know that I am not alone when I feel that everything is being speeded up for all of us. It's not just computers and electronics. From our metabolic rate to our ideas, we're processing things faster and faster. The time between understanding something and acting on that understanding is no longer spread over days and months. We're expected to react within moments. We are phoned, FedExed, and faxed much faster than our bodies and our minds or our spirits can respond. That's one of the primary reasons that it's so important that we stay connected to our core. This is the new destiny.

As we approach the year 2000, I'm convinced that those of us who will thrive in the new millennium are not necessarily those with the best résumés. Knowing how to use the newest version of Windows and knowing how to send info on the "Net" at the speed of light is not a sure prescription for success. Having a fax, a modem, a cellular phone, a high-speed computer, and a beeper may make you feel plugged in to the twenty-first century, but the only thing you may really be is wired. It is the people who are *internally* plugged in—the people who are most deeply connected to their inner selves and their spiritual guides—who will be the champions of the twenty-first century. This I am sure of.

Three days of fasting has brought you to a new beginning. It has given you a jump-start into a healthier, more connected life with a sense of your own inner being. Continue, embrace your lessons, and seek many more. Always seek more. You have already accomplished the most difficult task. You have started. You are blessed every day with the adventure and grace of life. When you are present to appreciate what is good and true, it will make itself available to you. Never be afraid. You are always in the right place at the right time, and you are always surrounded by abundance. That is your birthright. Give thanks to whatever power you believe has brought you here. Give thanks for this journey. Give of yourself and to yourself.

Appendix A

YOGA

Because yoga and detox go hand in hand so naturally, I've included ten basic yoga postures. These postures are an easy-to-use collection of exercises that cleanse, invigorate, and balance the system. These postures are my constant companions. I call them my spiritual "six-pack" because I always do at least six of them every day. Whether I'm traveling halfway around the world, or traveling from my kitchen to my bedroom. If I feel out of shape, I have my yoga; if I feel beaten up, I have my yoga; if I feel overwhelmed, I have my yoga; if I feel uncertain and alone, I have my yoga. I use yoga as a body-affirming method. I want you to have these same "friends" to always come home to during your three days of fasting—and beyond.

Legend has it that yoga evolved from the union of the healing arts and the martial arts, a process that began with Buddha and his epic journey. Stories tell us that this was all Buddha required for his travels through life. No coffeemaker, no blow-dryer, no magazines, and no Walkman—only the techniques that have come to be known as yoga. At the end of a yoga session, you typically feel a transcendence of your physical limitation of who you are to an enlightened state. It's a union with one's spiritual essence. That's quite an endorsement! No wonder that after 2,500 years, yoga is more popular than ever.

You don't *have* to practice yoga to have a successful detox. But it is very important to me that you have the option. Maybe you'll do these exercises only once or maybe you'll do them every day. That choice is yours. You don't need to begin these exercises now, but I would like you to try to imagine how soothing and supportive these different yoga exercises might feel when practiced during the fast.

Yoga Tips

- When you practice your yoga, I suggest that you do so on a mat or large towel (beach towel) for comfort and for traction.
- Look at the accompanying drawings, and follow the instructions for each pose as best you can.
- Never push your body too hard—that is totally contrary to the spirit of yoga.
- There are no hard and fast rules—only do what your body needs to do and is capable of doing.
- Always move slowly and deliberately, fully conscious of the exchange of breath inside you. Your positions will all evolve and strengthen with practice.
- Always be where your breath is; always have your breath move you. The more fully you breathe, the more each motion will come to life.
- Ideally these ten yoga exercises are best done in sequence. Doing them all as outlined should take you about fifteen minutes. If you don't have the time, of course, just do one or two.

The more you practice the following exercises the more you are going to wake up your body. Don't be surprised if you feel aches days later, or if you experience various telltale signs that a spontaneous cleansing is going on. Yoga will go through your body like a combustion—a light spearing through. And any place that is dark and dense will start to lighten up.

Yoga is all about oneness, bringing you out of your head and into your heart. Practice it regularly, and it will always bring you into truth and harmony.

EXERCISE #1: THE RAG DOLL AND THE SWEEP

Stand with your feet about three inches apart. Root yourself firmly into the ground, letting your heels and soles and toes plant flat on the floor. Feel the earth connect and imagine strong, sinewy roots grabbing you and growing up through your legs, through your spine, up your back, and through the top of your head. Raise your hands in the air, as high as you can reach, and stand very straight for a minute in this position. Feel the roots grow up through to the tips of your fingers. Now, relax completely at the waist and let the top half of your body gently fall forward, and over like a limp rag doll. Exhale fully as your body drops over, knees slightly bent. Let everything hang, completely relaxed. Breathe into the relaxation.

Now very slowly, vertebra by vertebra (lower vertebrae first), lift your body back up until you are once again fully upright in a perfect straight pose. Do this so slowly, like a puppet on a string, giving each vertebra of your spine a chance to connect and bring itself into beautiful alignment.

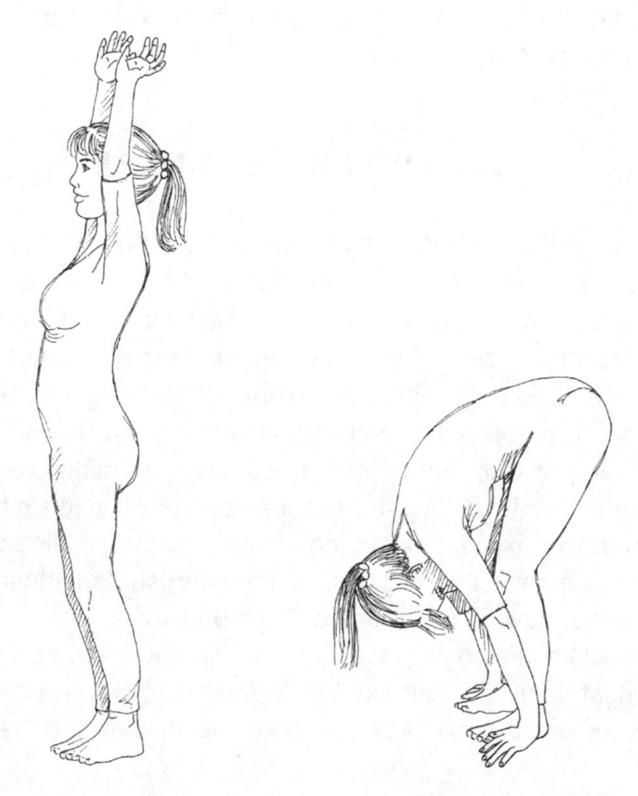

Move your feet two more inches apart. Put both of your arms straight out in front of you with the backs of your hands touching. You are going to create an imaginary circle by sweeping your arms away from each other, as though you are swimming and using the breaststroke. Sweep open a large circle with your arms, letting them carry all the way behind you. Let your palms touch behind your back if you can reach. If you can't get all the way there, just go back as far as you can. Keeping your hands behind you, palms touching if possible, relax once again at the waist and drop forward like a rag doll. Let your hands drop, then come back up slowly in the same way, one vertebra at a time.

Standing up straight again, cup your palms now and bring them both toward you as if you are bringing a big ball of light toward the center of the stomach. This is your vital energy. This motion should be done very, very, very slowly—really concentrating on what kind of energy you want inside of you. Let your cupped palms meet in the center of your stomach, still not quite touching. Now let them glide up and down your body, up and down over the legs, abdomen, chest, and shoulders like a protective coating. Finally, let them come to rest cupped over your eyes.

EXERCISE #2: THE TRIANGLE

Stand now with your feet wide apart, and once again root firmly into the ground. Extend your arms out fully in front of you and imagine that you are about to pull on two ropes. At the end of these two ropes is all the *prana* energy of the universe, all the oxygen and vital force your body could ever need, and I want you to bring it in. So imagine grabbing these ropes, one with each hand, and pull them toward you like in a tug of war. As you pull these ropes in, make a sound with your breath, a loud "Whoosh." Whoosh and pull it in. It's a tug-of-war with your own oxygen, extending your arms, then pulling them in to your waist, elbows bending, with a firm whoosh. Pull those ropes in, and pull that oxygen in ten times. Then pause.

Keeping your upright pose, turn your right foot out so it is pointing to the right, and turn your left foot slightly so it is also pointing right. Keep your entire torso facing forward, as though you were staring straight ahead. Extend your arms out at your sides, at shoulder height. Now, let the weight of your right arm tip you over toward your right side, bending at the hip, so that your right hand drops to your right ankle and your left hand rises to point palm-up at the sky. Your head also turns to face the sky. Breathe into your hips to make them flexible. Breathe into the pose.

Rise up slowly. You may feel some cracks. That's good. Face both feet forward and pause for a few moments. Come back to your center and regain your balance. Now point your left foot out to the left and turn your right foot slightly to the left. Keep your torso facing forward. Arms out to the sides, at shoulder height. Now reach over to the left side, dropping your left arm down toward the left ankle as your right arm rises up with your palm facing the sky. Your head should also rotate to face up at the sky. Breathe into your hips to loosen them; breathing all the time. After a few seconds in this position, rise up once again and come back to your center.

This is the Triangle, and in this exercise you're opening up your hips, your flexibility, and your ability to change. With flexibility, change can enter the body and be absorbed, keeping you free of illness and open to the future.

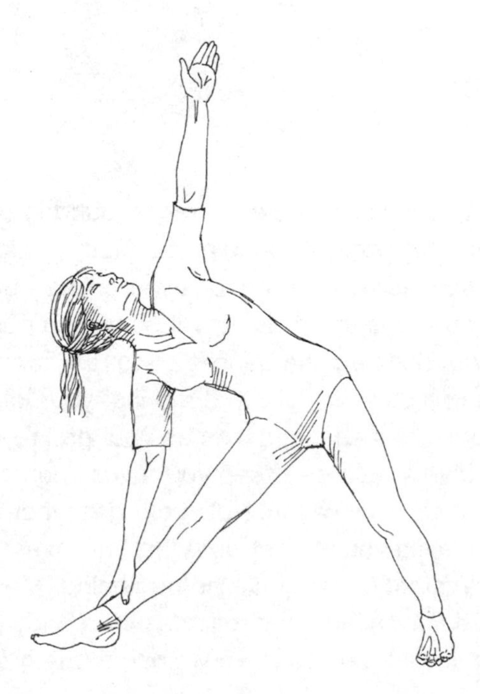

EXERCISE #3: THE TREE

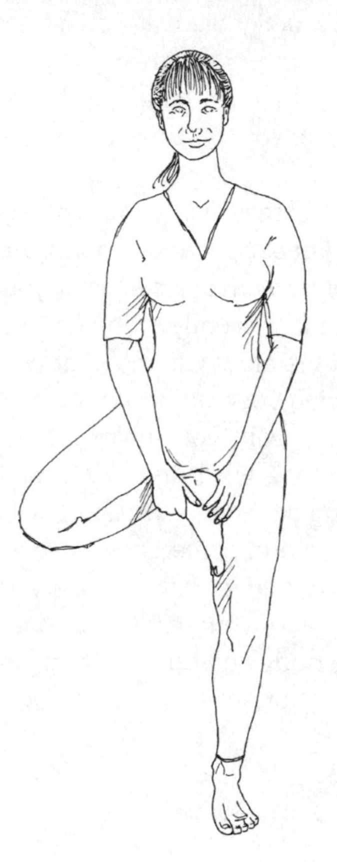

The Tree gives you a sense of being very grounded and connected to the earth. Start this pose by standing perfectly straight and getting rooted in both your legs. Focus your eyes on an object directly in front of you. Focusing is the "trick" in all balancing poses.

Now take your right leg and bend it up to rest comfortably off the ground. You can place your right foot against your left leg—on your left ankle, on your left knee, or as high as your groin—as high as you can and still hold your balance. Keep your eyes open and focused on something straight in front of you. Hold your gaze there, knowing that if you close your eyes you will get dizzy and fall over.

This posture might be tough in the beginning. Most of us are off balance a lot in our lives, and that reflects in the body. So if you have to, start with your right foot down very close to the ground, touching your left foot at the bottom of your ankle if necessary, and center yourself there. As you get more comfortable and confident, you will be able to raise your leg to a higher position. If you start to wobble, strengthen your focus.

Once you are standing on one leg, cup both palms of your hands together, in a prayer position, and hold them over your head. Remain in this position for two or three minutes if possible.

Standing on both legs again, pause for a few minutes to restabilize yourself, and then repeat this exercise lifting your left leg this time. Hold the position for several minutes and feel the balance. Then replant your left foot on the ground.

EXERCISE #4: THE CAT POSE

This position begins with you on your knees, your toes dug into the floor for rooting. Take both of your hands now, opening them up as flat and as wide as you can, and place them on the floor firmly, palms down, shoulder-width apart, like an animal on all fours. Open them even wider now as you dig them into the mat or towel you are practicing on. Allow your palms to sink into the ground so that you are firmly rooted in this position, arms comfortably forward.

From this position, let your stomach sink and fall toward the ground and let your back fall with it, forming a curve. At the very same time, arch your neck up to the ceiling. Head and neck up, stomach and back dropped. Use your arms for support, keeping them close to the body, with your elbows slightly bent. Inhale—a deep inhale. And hold this position for a moment. Now invert the pose. Curve your back up, like a cat walking across a fence. Arch your back like a Halloween black cat, pull your stomach into the body, and let your head drop toward the ground. Exhale fully.

Once again now, pull your head and neck up to the sky and let your stomach and back drop in a beautiful curve, approaching the ground. Inhale. Then it's head down, back way up in a beautiful arch, stomach curled, exhale. That's the Cat Pose, wonderful for balancing the body.

Remaining on all fours, turn your head and look all the way to the left hip. Stretch yourself open. Now turn your head the other way,

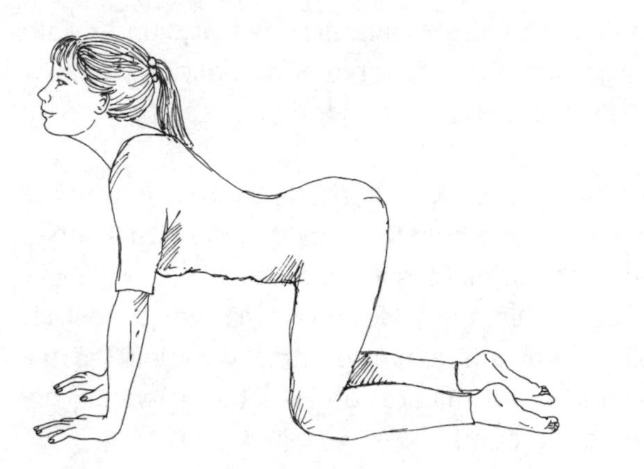

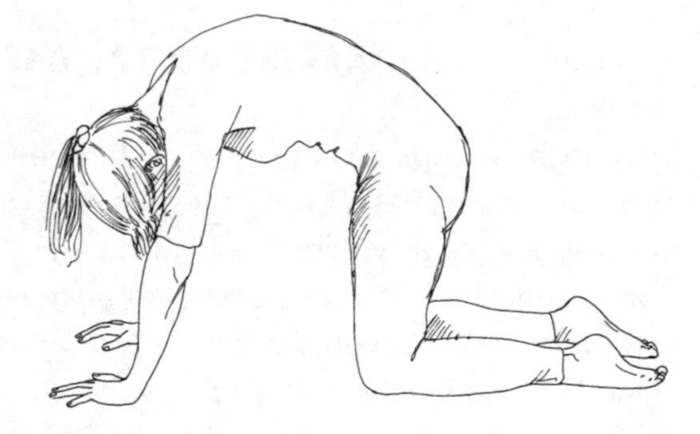

looking all the way to the
right hip. More stretch. Then come back to center.

EXERCISE #5: THE DOWNWARD DOG

Start in the all-fours position, on your hands and knees, with your toes tucked under and your hands slightly forward in the Cat Pose. Turn your head down now and slowly straighten your knees, using the power of the thighs, raising your butt high into the air. Let your toes prop you up in the air so that your butt is higher than any other part of you. You're off your heels now, letting your feet stretch from heel to toe, taking deep easy breaths and feeling the stretch in your hamstrings. Stay in this position for several minutes. This is the Downward Dog.

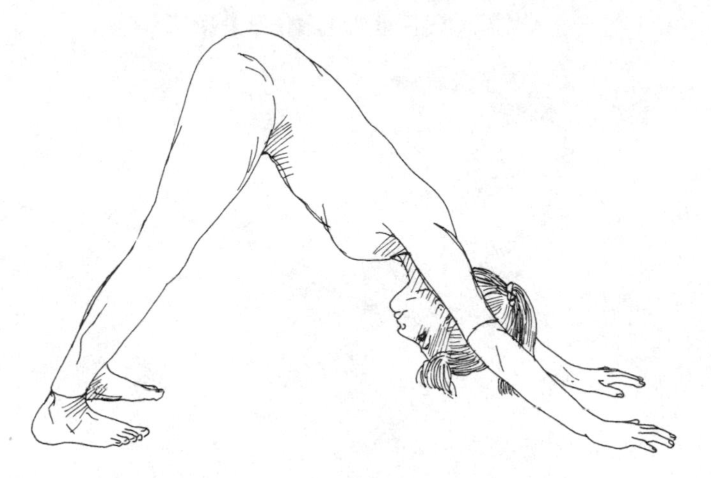

EXERCISE #6: THE COBRA

This is a wonderful way to strengthen the muscles of your back and stomach. Start by lying on the floor facedown, palms flat on the floor at each shoulder, your elbows bent and close to your body, and your forehead touching the ground. Now inhale while you use your stomach and back muscles to raise your chest off the ground. Use your arms only for support. Feel the strength in your spine. Stretch your head and look at the ceiling as you arch your spine backward as far as you can without coming off the ground.

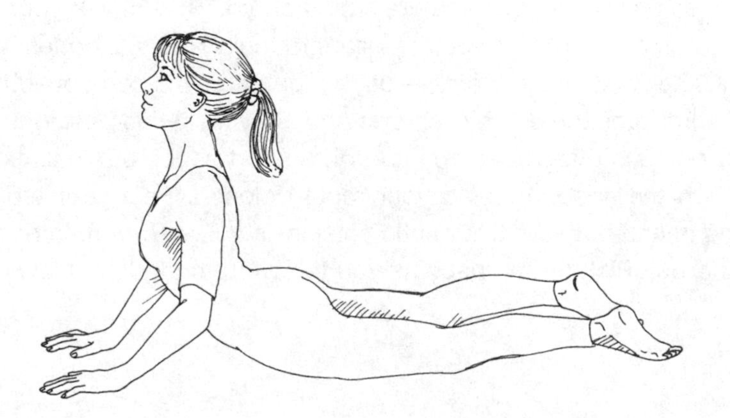

EXERCISE #7: CHILD POSE

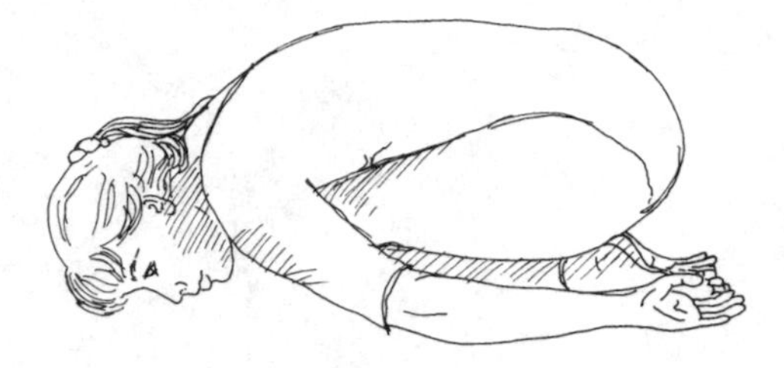

Moving out of the Cobra pose, relax now, rising back onto all fours. Let your butt drop so that it is resting on your heels. Relax the rest of your body so that your chest drops to your knees and your forehead drops till it is lightly resting on the floor. You can put your hands straight in front of you or relaxed by your sides, whichever feels most comfortable. Rest in this position taking deep easy breaths. This is the Child Pose. It's like a child resting; a complete womblike state, where you can safely reconnect to the center of your energy. Rest here for at least two or three minutes.

Rise up now so that you are sitting on your heels with your torso upright. Make sure that your heels are touching the sitz bones, which are at the point just at the base of your behind. This contact activates and stimulates the energy centers. And, staying in this position, place both palms on your stomach and do a short series of small exhales through the nose, keeping your mouth closed. Feel your stomach going in and out with this gentle version of a Fire Breath. In and out. In and out. Pick up the pace as you feel more confident. Now rest.

EXERCISE #8: THE EGG

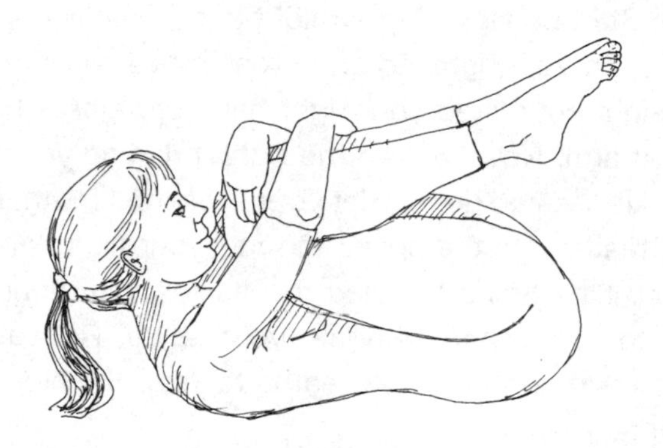

Start by lying comfortably on your back, legs and arms comfortably extended. Bring your knees up to your chest and hold them close with both arms in a firm hug. Gently rock back and forth in this position. Give yourself a good hug and give your back a good stretch as you open your spine up through this rocking motion. So many of us feel unsupported in life, and that can translate into back spasms and discomfort. Feel your back supported by the earth now, and feel yourself being supported by its strength and power. If you have a lullaby, now is a good time to sing it as you rock back and forth, stretching and strengthening. This is known as The Egg Pose, so think of it as a way to coddle yourself.

EXERCISE # 9: THE SPINAL TWIST

This exercise is a good way to increase flexibility and relieve pressure in the spine. Start by sitting up straight and stretching your legs out again. Now bend your right leg and cross it over your left leg (which remains straight out); keep your right hand straight behind you and raise your left arm. Now twist to the right, bringing your left hand to your right ankle. As you do this, let your eyes travel with the full range of motion. Breathe into the pose, and feel your hips doing the work. Opening your hips helps to open the flexibility of your body. Now come back to center and elongate your spine. Repeat on the left side, always taking deep, easy breaths to keep the hips loose. Then return to center.

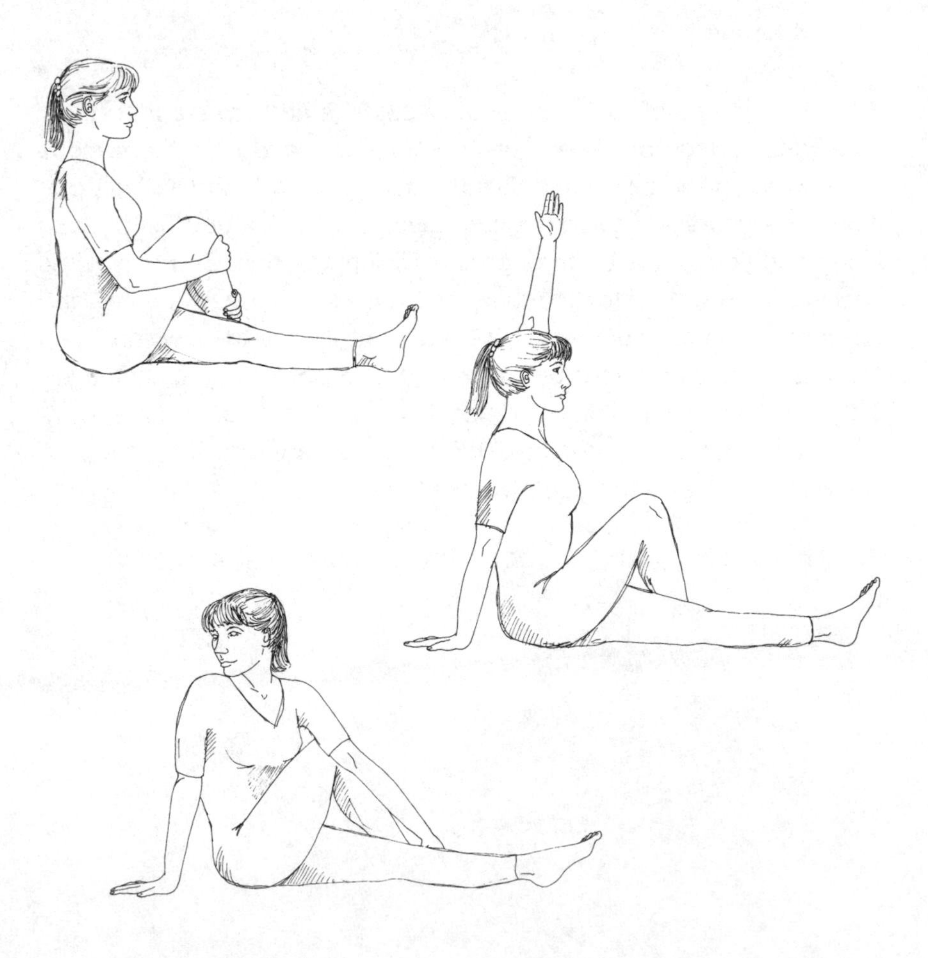

EXERCISE #10: FINAL STRETCH AND SQUAT

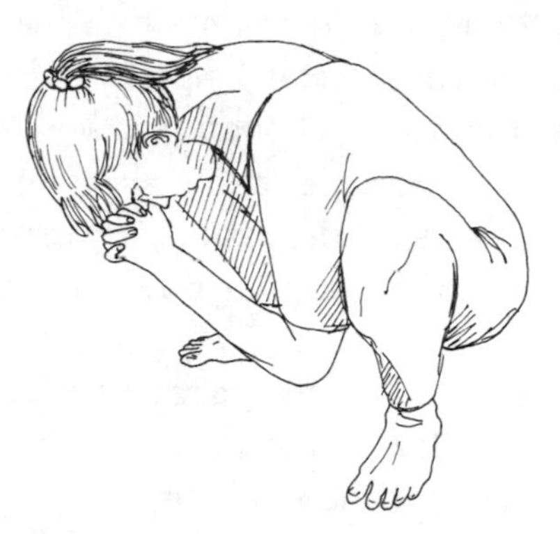

Sometimes we squat for comfort. Sometimes we squat for rest. Sometimes we squat to get down, get real, and touch the earth. And sometimes we squat because we can't find a bench. But squatting is also a quick, simple, highly effective way to ward off one of the unpleasant side effects of fasting: light-headedness.

Some people will get light-headed periodically during their days of fasting. If you don't want to lie down, or you can't lie down, squatting is your best medicine. Squatting lets you draw energy from the earth to balance you and center you; it fills you with an immediate sense of groundedness and connection. It's powerful stuff, and you can use it as often as you need it.

Whether or not you are experiencing lightheadedness during the fast, I encourage you to drop to the ground in a squat several times a day and let yourself feel closer to the earth for a few minutes. Why? Because to me, squatting is more than a simple exercise; being grounded is a beautiful metaphor for letting Mother Nature and her earth energy provide for you and nurture you. Getting more connected to your insides also means getting more connected to the earth that supports you, and nothing makes that connection faster than squatting.

Whether you are working through a single pose, or a long routine, this final rooting exercise is a valuable way to complete your daily yoga work.

Start by going to any wall in your room. Facing the wall, extend your arms in front of you at shoulder height, out to the wall, and press your palms against the wall as though you were making two handprints. Now, slowly step both feet back, away from the wall, and let your back sink in as your shoulders squeeze together. Keep it gentle, like a little massage moving up and down the spine between the shoulders.

Stand up now, turn around, and get straight up against the wall—really straight and tall. Slowly drop at the waist and try to reach as low as you can with your hands, reaching toward your toes. Keep your butt firmly pressed against the wall and your legs straight. Breathe deeply and really feel your hamstrings stretch. Feel yourself completely in your body, in the union that is yoga. You are where you need to be.

Slowly come back up, straight back up against the wall. Move a few steps away from the wall, plant your feet shoulder-width apart, clasp your hands together in a prayer pose, and squat down to the ground. Squat down and rest on your haunches. Imagine now roots coming up through the ground and into your body—coming up through your feet, through your calves, through your thighs, through your belly, through your chest, through your neck, and through your head. Imagine those roots now growing up through the top of your head and into the heavens. Let heaven and earth connect you and everything. Let heaven and earth connect all your actions, and all your thoughts. And now let your butt drop completely to the ground so that you are sitting cross-legged or in a position that feels comfortable. Relax. Breathe fully. Draw an imaginary circle of white light around yourself as you sit in this position. Let the circle be your protection for the day. Keep this circle around you so that everything that is supposed to be in your sphere will be, and nothing else will intrude. Then raise both palms up, pressed together in the prayer pose, and bring them to touch your face in the "third eye" space right between your eyes. Softly say, "Namaste," which means, "I honor the light within you." Now fall into the deepest part of yourself as you prepare to move naturally into the rooting ritual.

ROOTING RITUAL
TO COMPLETE YOGA SESSION

From a standing position, relax your knees and let your body slowly drop to the ground until you are resting comfortably on your haunches in the squat position. Let yourself relax fully, and let your weight press you firmly into the earth. Clasp your hands in front of you, almost as though you were in prayer, and use them to help you stay balanced. If you discover that this basic positioning is uncomfortable, try to find your own comfortable position that makes you feel as close to the ground as possible.

The earth has endured for millions of years. It has endured through hurricanes, blizzards, tornadoes, and earthquakes. And it continues to renew itself. Still, every spring we're genuinely surprised by the amount of life it gives forth. And every autumn we're amazed by how it takes us into its beauty before it turns inward for winter. The earth, in its cycles, is a source of continuity, strength, sustenance, solace, and spiritual attunement. And it is in this place you want to connect now.

In your squatting position, feel the strength and weight of the earth beneath you. Now imagine that strength moving up through your feet and legs, and into the center of your body where your vital force is strongest. Feel that strength and weight as they move through your body to the center. Feel their simplicity. Feel their aliveness. Feel their power.

Now ask the earth to replenish you—to replenish the sides of you that have been too high in the air, too much in the mind, and too removed from the body. You want to come back into the most grounded form, your basic nature. Let it help you connect to your deepest nature, that wants to be still, that wants to be compassionate, that wants to be kind. Ask the earth to help you come back into the place of beauty, where your flowers are always seeding, where the body is always coming forth with new life. Then ask that the wisdom of nature take over, and allow the cycles of nature to flow through you without interference from your mind and your will.

As you allow these greater forces to move through you from the earth, allow yourself now to plant something in this ritual. It doesn't matter what it is you plant. It doesn't have to be tangible. It can be an idea. A hope. A wish. A seed. A home. A relationship. Imagine yourself planting, and dig your hands into the earth. Feel the ground and the mud mineralizing you, stabilizing you, and rooting you. Feel the ground keeping you from running off to yet another place, keeping you focused and keeping you still.

In this rooted place, everything begins to grow and flower. It is time to feel that root grow. Feel that root coming up your spine, growing like branches through your spine, your ribs, your kidneys, your pancreas, your arms, your legs, your neck, your shoulders, your ears, your eyes, and your hair. Feel it going right up through you—growing right up through you. And now feel how deeply connected you are to the earth—attached to the earth—one with the earth.

Appendix B

RECIPES

With all of the following juices, use your own judgment about the ingredients. If you know, for example, that ginger upsets your stomach, don't include it. The amount of juice you will get depends on the size and ripeness of the fruit or vegetable. Don't be afraid to compensate for produce variations by doubling up on the ingredients. Most of these juices have a really rich taste and can be diluted with a little bit of springwater. If you find that any of them tastes too sweet or too strong, use water to cut the taste.

These recipes should deliver a really generous amount of juice. If you don't immediately finish it, use the leftover juice for snacking. Something to remember: Although fresh is always better, you can freeze fruit juice; but you don't want to freeze vegetable juice. (For tips on selecting and prepping your fruits and vegetables, see pages 244–46.)

MORNING DRINK (PINAPPLE-PAPAYA-STRAWBERRY)

½ pineapple, peeled
½ papaya or 1 mango, peeled, seeds or pits removed

4–8 strawberries, tops removed
2 tablespoons flaxseed oil (refrigerated)
1 tablespoon acidophilus (refrigerated)
2 cups water
1 cup mango or papaya juice (if available)

Take half a pineapple and cut it up into small pieces. Take half a papaya, scoop out and discard the seeds. Put this fruit in your blender, along with a handful of strawberries. Add the flaxseed oil, acidophilus, water, and mango or papaya juice (if available), and blend thoroughly. I like my morning drink rich and thick so I can really feel the weight of the fruits in my mouth when I drink. If you prefer a thinner drink, add more water. If you can't find mango or papaya juice, add more of the other fruit. Keep anything you don't drink in the refrigerator for an anytime pick-me-up. (The morning drink is the only one you make in your blender.)

APPLE-STRAWBERRY-GRAPE

2–3 medium-sized apples (preferably Red Delicious)
6 strawberries
2 cups red seedless grapes

Cut the apples into small sections that fit easily into your juicer, removing the core and seeds; remove the tops from the strawberries, and pick off all stems from the grapes. Start by juicing the strawberries and grapes in your juicer. Then juice all the apples.

APPLE-PEAR-GINGER

6 Red Delicious apples
4 brown pears
1 nickel-sized piece of ginger (optional)

Cut the apples and pears into small sections and remove the core and seeds before putting in juicer with ginger (optional).

CARROT-BEET-APPLE

8–10 large juicing carrots
½ large red beet
1 large Red Delicious apple
1 nickel-sized piece of ginger (optional)

Juice the apple first. Next, juice the carrots and the beet (you can include the top of the beet, if you wish). For an extra rev of energy, juice the ginger as well, but only if you know your stomach can handle it. Stir.

CABBAGE-CARROT-CELERY

¼ head of cabbage
8 carrots
2 stalks celery
½ Red Delicious apple

Core the apple, and juice all the ingredients.

GRAPE JUICE

Let your own eyes control the amount of grapes you need. Water should be added to this drink because it's so strong and sweet. The measurements are 3 parts grape juice to 1 part water.

2 (approximately) big bunches of grapes
water

GREEN VEGETABLE DRINK

½ head of cabbage
3 stalks celery
1 handful parsley

1 handful (bunch) kale
1 handful spinach
1 cucumber, peeled
1 apple

Don't be afraid to be creative with this juice. If you feel like adding other ingredients like fennel, green pepper, or romaine, do so. If it feels as though you are juicing the whole farm, then you've captured the feeling. For additional liver cleansing, add a clove of garlic.

PINEAPPLE-PEAR-LEMON

½ pineapple, peeled
1½ pears (I use the Bosc variety for this juice)
½ lemon
1 nickel-sized piece of ginger (optional)

Cut up the pineapple and put in juicer, followed by the pears and ginger (if your stomach can handle it). Pour into a glass and add the lemon juice.

PINEAPPLE-ORANGE-STRAWBERRY

1 pineapple, peeled
1½ oranges, peeled, seeded
2 handfuls strawberries (about 10 berries)

Cut up the pineapple and orange and put through juicer along with the berries.

This juice will keep for twenty-four hours in the refrigerator as long as you shake it regularly.

CARROT-CABBAGE-APPLE

8 carrots
¼ head of cabbage
1½ Red Delicious apple

Core and cut up the apple, and juice all the ingredients.

ORGANIC MARY

4 or 5 medium-sized tomatoes
3 large ribs celery
1 medium-sized red pepper
1 nickel-sized piece of horseradish
touch of tamari

Juice all of the vegetables and the horseradish, and blend together to desired thickness, adding a touch of tamari.

WARM VEGETABLE BROTH

Store the remaining broth in the refrigerator, and reheat it each night on the stove top. Do not use a microwave oven, since it is likely to rob your broth of many of its essential nutrients.

1 medium-sized head of cabbage
3 large red beets
3 medium-sized potatoes
1 large green onion (or 2 small ones)
1 head of parsley
4 cloves of garlic
6 large carrots
2 stalks celery
½ butternut squash (scoop out seeds)
2 twigs fresh thyme
dash of tamari
water to cover

I like to cook the broth in a giant stockpot so the ingredients have room to mix and interact. If you don't have a giant pot, it's okay to use two, or even three, smaller pots, but make sure the ingredients are not so squashed together that you cannot stir them.

Put all of your ingredients into the pot(s). If you have other vegetables such as broccoli, spinach, or zucchini (organic, please) sitting in your refrigerator, this is the perfect time to clean your refrigerator out and add these ingredients to the mix. Next, pour in fresh water—the purest available—till the waterline rises half an inch above all of the vegetables. Bring this giant collection of nature's best to a boil, cover your pot, and keep it at a low boil for at least twenty-five minutes. Turn off the heat and let it sit for another fifteen to twenty minutes. Strain the broth and discard all of the vegetable remains, thanking them for their contribution of vitamins, minerals, and exceptional flavor. I often mash the cooked carrots and squash and give them to my dog as a special treat.

DESSERT DRINKS

MANGO-PEACH-GINGER

5 or 6 mangoes
2 medium-sized peaches
1 slice of lime (optional)
1 nickel-sized piece of ginger (optional)

Peel the mango, and remove the pit or stone. Take the pits out of the peaches. Cut up the fruit and put in juicer along with the ginger, if your stomach can handle it. Pour into glass and add a slice of lime. This is really nice on hot summer days.

BERRY COBBLER

6 Red Delicious or Granny Smith Apples (if you like a tart juice)
1 handful blueberries

1 handful raspberries
1 handful strawberries
1 sprig of mint (optional)
½ lime

Core and cut up the apples, and juice the fruit and the mint. Pour into a glass and add the juice from ½ lime.

GREEN APPLE-CUCUMBER DRINK

4 medium-sized green apples
1½ cucumbers, peeled

Core the apple before putting it and the sliced cucumber in your juicer.

PINEAPPLE-CUCUMBER DRINK

½ pineapple
1 large cucumber, peeled

Slice the pineapple and cucumber and put in your juicer.

REMEDIES TO THE RESCUE

Some people sail through their fasting days with only the minimum amount of discomfort. Others go through the process a little bit worried about how their bodies might surprise them. Still others may experience mild sequential discomforts as various toxins make their exits. The best defense against today's anxieties and "complications," as I like to call them, is knowing how to prepare a medicine cabinet full of juice remedies that can be at your disposal within minutes.

Look up and down this list. You don't have to make any of these remedy juices, but you should know that you *can* make them at any time. Most people find that these great juices are very helpful. If you discover that you have only a small portion of juice with some of these recipes, don't think you made a mistake.

For **headaches**, try juicing three large Granny Smith apples and adding a pinch of sea salt.

For **light-headedness**, try juicing 5 carrots, 2 stalks of celery, ½ apple, 2 handfuls of parsley, and 3 leaves of kale. This juice acts like two strong arms holding you upright and steady.

For **constipation** combine the juice of 2 handfuls of spinach and 4 carrots. Or, for another sweeter, gentler approach to this common Day 2 dilemma, juice 3 apples, 1 pear, and a tiny piece of ginger.

The onset of **menstrual cramps** can be soothed with the juice of ½ head of cabbage combined with the juices of 2 stalks of celery, a handful of parsley, and a 2-inch piece of fennel.

Feeling **nervous**? Try juicing 8 carrots and 2 stalks of celery.

Remember that the idea here is to open yourself up to a new approach to wellness, and avoid conventional treatments like over-the-counter drugs and hard-core prescription medication if at all possible. You might discover that these simple, and often scrumptious, natural remedies work so well that you will clean out the contents of your medicine cabinet and follow the natural road from now on.

A WORD ABOUT ORGANIC PRODUCE

The fruits and vegetables you use for this program must be fresh and, whenever possible, they should be organically grown. Organic produce may be a little bit more expensive, but I think it's an expense that is well worth it. Most nonorganic supermarket produce is coated with beeswax, a food-grade vegetable petroleum, or sometimes even a shellac-based wax or resin to maintain freshness. It makes those huge piles of "fresh" produce look more like wax-museum sculpture than nature's bounty. And these treatments don't come off with just a good rinse in the sink. It's scary enough to make you scream.

And then there is the problem of herbicides, pesticides, and "etcetera-icides"—all of that frightening stuff that you're trying to get *out* of your body through fasting. The last thing you need to be doing is putting more bad stuff in right now. The 3-Day Ultimate Detox is about giving yourself a "fresh start," and that should start with fresh, organically grown produce. These days, no one needs to travel very far to find organic produce. You can find it at many supermarkets, most health-food stores, food co-ops, farm stands, and farmer's markets. If you aren't sure that it is certified organic, ask before you buy.

Personally, I think organic produce always tastes better and tastes fresher. It really tastes more *alive*. Don't be surprised to discover that once you've gone organic you may not want to go back to conventional produce.

Here are a few more helpful hints:

PINEAPPLES: The pineapple is ripe when the "leaves" can be easily plucked from the top and it smells sweet. Start by cutting off the crown at least one inch below the point where the leaves meet the top of the fruit. Cut off at least one-half inch from the bottom. Fully peel the remaining pineapple. Cut the remaining fruit into quarters, and then into smaller wedges. Make sure the wedges are small enough to fit easily into your *blender*.

APPLES: Organic apples do not have to be skinned before juicing. Remove any stems, then quarter your apples. Now cut out all of the pips (apple pips can be mildly toxic, and I would prefer it if you wouldn't juice them). Because apples leave a lot of pulp that can quickly clog up the juicer, I always juice my apples separately from other fruits. Green apples juice up the best. Red Delicious apples also juice up well. Mealy, overripe apples do not juice well.

STRAWBERRIES: Pick the green tops off. Wash them especially thoroughly—strawberry skin holds on to dirt. If your strawberries are white at the top, cut that top portion off.

PAPAYA: Peel the papaya completely. Next, cut it in half and remove all of the black seeds from the middle with a clean spoon. Discard these seeds (or plant them). Finally, cut the papaya in quarters.

GRAPES: Pick all of your grapes off their stems, then wash the grapes thoroughly. Do not juice the stems.

PEARS: Organic pears do not have to be skinned, but they do need to be washed thoroughly. Remove the stems. Cut into quarters and remove all of the pips. You want your pears to be ripe, but still firm. Overripe pears do not juice well, and yield very little juice.

MANGO: Peel away and discard the mango skin. Cut mango in half at the center around the large nut and peel away fleshy fruit from the nut. (Discard or plant the nut.) Cut fleshy fruit into several smaller pieces.

WATERMELON: Do not juice the rind. Remove as many seeds as possible before juicing.

CARROTS: Organic carrots do not need to be peeled, but they do need to be washed thoroughly. Heavy-duty juicers can juice carrots whole. For other juicers, slice carrots in half lengthwise, then into quarters. Cut into smaller pieces if necessary.

GREENS: Wash all greens thoroughly before juicing.

POTATOES, BEETS, AND OTHER VEGGIES: Most organic produce does not have to be peeled before juicing or boiling, but the skins do need to be scrubbed thoroughly to remove residual dirt and fertilizer.

GARLIC: Separate cloves and remove all exterior skin before juicing or boiling.

NOTE: Although we advise you not to *eat* fruits and vegetables together, many *juice* combinations are okay because they don't require mixing enzymes for digestion.

Appendix C

MY TOP TEN: MUSIC FOR THE SPIRITUAL LIBRARY

Healing by Spiritual Environment
Shamanic Dream by Spiritual Environment
Migration by Peter Kater and Carlos Nakai
Ritual by Gabriel Roth
Chant (CD) by the Benedictine Monks of Santo Domingo de Silos
Soundtrack to *Out of Africa*
Jiva Mukti by Nada Shakti and Bruce Becvar
Singing Stones (CD) by Michael Stearns and Ron Sunsinger
Phantasys by Danny Wright
Shepherd Moons by Enya

MY TOP TEN: BOOKS FOR THE SPIRITUAL LIBRARY

Care of the Soul by Thomas Moore
The Alchemist by Paulo Coelho
Seat of the Soul by Gary Zucker
The Way of the Peaceful Warrior by Dan Melman

Autobiography of a Yogi by Krishnamurti
Spontaneous Healing by Andrew Weil, M.D.
The Seven Spiritual Laws of Success by Deepak Chopra
Staying Healthy with the Seasons by Elmore Haas
Spiritual Emergency by Stanislav Groff
Joy's Way by Brough Joy